"THE PILL"

"THE PILL"

By Morton Mintz

AN ALARMING REPORT

Beacon Press   Boston

For Margaret, Roberta, and Daniel

Acknowledgments

My thanks go first of all to the editors of the *Washington Post* who have given a too often obstreperous reporter the indispensable support he needed to try to penetrate the arcane mysteries of The Pill.

In addition to the *Washington Post,* my thanks go also to those others for whom I have written, in different form, much of the material in this book: Houghton Mifflin Co., publisher of my book *The Therapeutic Nightmare* (1965); Beacon Press, publisher of *By Prescription Only* (1967), which HMCo. issued in hardcover; the National Catholic Features Co-operative, the *New Republic,* and *Columbia Journalism Review.*

The newspaper, the books, the magazines, the readers, and I—all were at the receiving end. There were several people at the giving end—men who took risks and who sacrificed greatly of their time and energy to help me get the facts out. They were serving the public interest—your interest—and not their self-interest. That distinguishes them from many of the persons you will encounter in this book. Some of my sources cannot be named. One in particular: without him, a brave, brilliant, and dedicated public servant, I would not have gotten The Pill story very far off the ground.

I want to express my deep gratitude and admiration to Dr. Herbert Ratner, a profound and wise human being and a great physician, who as long ago as 1962 put together a prescient list of troublesome questions about The Pill. He is a most active and busy man, being, among other things, health director of the Village of Oak Park, Illinois. Yet he has found time to edit *Child and Family* and, incredibly, to assemble for each issue "A Sampler on The Pill," which has drawn on a wide range of sources to bring together in a single place summaries of what is being written about The Pill. To my knowledge, this obvious and invaluable service is performed by no one in Government or anywhere else. Dr. Ratner's "Samplers" were invaluable in the writing of this book.

Finally, I thank my wife Anita for helping me and sustaining me in a strenuous period.

MORTON MINTZ

Washington, D.C.
August 1969

Contents

"THE PILL"

Introduction

"If I had a daughter who was about to marry, and if she were to ask what I believe to be the factual truth about contraceptive methods, this is what I would tell her." This was the way I began "One Father's Advice," an article published on March 26, 1967, in a special *Brides* supplement to *Potomac,* the Sunday magazine of the *Washington Post.* I wrote the article at the request of Walter H. Pincus, the then editor of *Potomac,* who suggested that it would be useful to distill the reporting I had done on The Pill since 1962 into a combination narrative and practical guide for girls and women concerned about contraception. In the more than two years since the article appeared I have kept up with developments involving The Pill and have written extensively about it—mainly in the *Washington Post;* in my book *By Prescription Only* (1967), which was a 60,000-word updating of *The Therapeutic Nightmare;* in the *New Republic,* and in the *Columbia Journalism Review.*

As in "One Father's Advice," I want to make a few things clear at once:

First, you will not find any preaching or even any discussion in this book about the religious and moral aspects of using The Pill—a contraceptive method that most probably prevents conception by suppressing ovulation; I am happy to leave that subject to others. My concern here is with the origins, development, and consequences of a fantastic medical experiment in which millions of women who are healthy—not sick—swallow powerful drugs 20 or 21 days a month.

Second, I have no personal, moral, or religious "hang-ups" about The Pill or about contraception generally. In fact, because of a long-standing concern about the problems of world population, my wife and I joined Planned Parenthood many years ago.

Third, the bulk of my reporting about The Pill has been focused on whether or not the presumed safety of The Pill had been demonstrated in advance of mass use. Nothing could have

pleased me more than to have found that The Pill was free of
hazards. However, the answers made it overwhelmingly clear
that safety had *not* been established.

Fourth, the hazards with which I am concerned here are
serious ones affecting health and life itself, not transient side
effects of The Pill such as nausea.

Fifth, safety is a *relative,* not an absolute, concept. This
cannot be too strongly emphasized. One must always ask,
"safe for whom?" One must always consider the ratio of benefit to risk. One must always understand that no drug is perfectly safe—that safety varies with the individual, with the
severity of his condition, with his age, with the reliability
with which he takes his medicine as the doctor ordered.
Water, salt, and sugar are staples of our diet but even they,
under certain circumstances, can cause serious disorders and
aggravate existing ones. In the case of The Pill, the essential
point in avoiding confusion is to shun talk about "women,"
because they are individual human beings and not a monolith; unlike guinea pigs in a medical laboratory, they vary im-
mensely one from the other. One who talks about "women"
can make generalizations about the safety of The Pill, and
these usually have a reassuring sound. But what do the generalizations have to do with you or your daughter or your sister
or your friend? The short answer is, not much. The oral contraceptives that combine an estrogen and a progestogen
(these and other medical terms are defined in the Glossary)
approach 100 percent efficacy in preventing conception. Thus
they may be relatively safe for the woman in whom conception could have tragic result—a death in childbirth, a mental
collapse, the birth of a child destined to starve or to deprive
older brothers and sisters of desperately needed food—because in her case efficacy is inseparable from safety. But can
it be truly said that The Pill, with all the risks cataloged in
this book, is relatively safe for a young suburban housewife
who wants a child but not just yet, especially if she could reliably use another form of effective contraception?

Sixth, there has been a lot of talk to the effect that—as
Helen Gurley Brown, editor of *Cosmopolitan* and author of
Sex and the Single Girl, has put it—The Pill "makes women
more desirous. Girls tell me they feel more sexy—they have
more energy in their viscera. It liberates a woman in bed."
Girls don't tell *me* that they feel more—or less—sexy on The
Pill, but I'd like to pass along to you what was said on this

point in *The Consumers Union Report on Family Planning,* which was prepared by the editors of *Consumer Reports* with the help of consultants who are very kindly disposed toward The Pill: "Although the pills seem to have no direct effect on sexual desire, in some field trials, among women who had constantly feared pregnancy, the reassurance of using an effective contraceptive caused two out of five participants to report an increase in sexual desire. On the other hand, a small number of women consistently find their libido diminished while taking oral contraceptives. It is impossible to say whether their problem is chemical or psychological in origin. . . . If sexual desire continues to be lessened, the woman is advised to try some other method of contraception." In a survey conducted in 1967 among 6733 physicians of the American College of Obstetricians and Gynecologists, 31 percent of those polled blamed The Pill for a decrease in the libido of their patients; 24 percent reported an increase. Three years ago at a marriage seminar in Kansas City, Missouri, Dr. William Masters, co-author with Virginia Johnson of *Human Sexual Response,* said that the first question to ask of a patient referred to a clinic for frigidity is, "Has she been taking The Pill?" Frigidity in women on The Pill, he continued, is "prevalent enough to make us suspicious when someone develops lack of responsiveness after taking it when she had been responsive before." The *Insiders' Newsletter for Women* of May 30, 1966, which reported Dr. Masters' remarks, also said that the same seminar was told by Dr. J. E. Eichenlaub of Minneapolis, that "Birth control pills, which spread progesterone action through the system during the entire month, play havoc with [woman's] sexual responsiveness." Dr. Michael Grounds reported in the *Medical Journal of Australia* for April 13, 1968, that loss of libido is "the commonest reason" for ceasing use of The Pill. "When this symptom is overlooked, the patient often develops a frank depressive state." In the same month Dr. Wade Cline said in *Davis' Gynecology and Obstetrics,* "A female chimpanzee given adequate estrogen will accept any male; however, following an injection of progesterone she rejects all males completely."

Seventh, there is heavy promotion to physicians of sequential forms of The Pill (C-Quens, Ortho-Novum SQ, Oracon, Norquen). Instead of taking a combination tablet on each of 20 days, a woman on a sequential regimen takes an estrogen tablet on some of those days and an estrogen/progestogen tablet on the other days. The risks are no less. The late Gregory Pincus, a co-discoverer of The Pill, was quoted in *The New York Times Magazine* in April 1966 as saying, "I see absolutely no advantage in the sequentials." However, they have a serious *disadvantage* that is not widely known. Women on the sequentials are taking risks that apparently are every bit as serious as those associated with the combinations but they are not getting the same high level of protection against becoming pregnant. According to the pro-Pill Dr. Robert W. Kistner (who blames failures on the fact that some women neglect to take one or two tablets in a 20- or 21-day cycle), users of the sequentials conceive at a rate of up to 5 percent per year. Dr. Christopher Tietze, of the Population Council, said last December 1 in *Ob. Gyn. News,* "The true failure rate could be as high as 10 pregnancies per 100 women per year."

Much reporting on The Pill has ignored the lesser efficacy of the sequentials. A classic example was provided in "The Week in Review" section of *The New York Times* on January 7, 1968. Jane E. Brody, then the *Times* specialist on The Pill, spoke of it in her first sentence as the "perfect" contraceptive; in her second she indicated that "perfect" had nothing to do with safety but was synonomous with "foolproof." Shooting the mother might also provide "perfect" contraception. In failing to distinguish between the almost 100 percent efficacy of the combinations and the lesser reliability of the sequentials, Miss Brody must have been unaware of a lawsuit filed a month before by Mrs. Jane Losh of Withamsville, Ohio. While on a sequential, she became pregnant with her seventh child.

Dr. Louis M. Hellman, chairman of the Advisory Committee on Obstetrics and Gynecology of the Food and Drug Administration, has consistently downgraded the reliability of the diaphragm by indicating its rate of failure in preventing conception to be about 10 percent.[1] Dr. Kistner has used a 12 percent rate. Yet, according to one careful study, the failure rate is much less, between 2.9 and 4.5 percent. Many authorities think the true rate is far lower. For example, Dr. Waldo L. Fielding, assistant professor of obstetrics and gyne-

[1] Dr. Hellman did this, for example, in a signed article in *Redbook* for April 1969, in which he said flatly that "the diaphragm has a 10 percent failure rate," and in an interview with C. P. Gilmore for an article on July 20, 1969, in *The New York Times Magazine.*

cology at the Tufts and Boston University medical schools, has put the rate at "less than 1 percent." The explanation for such seemingly irreconcilable figures is simple and important. The rates in the high range of failure are for, or include, poorly motivated women who are forgetful, careless, or otherwise unreliable and inconsistent in using a diaphragm. The failure rate is very low, approaching that of the combination Pill, for women who consistently use a diaphragm and use it properly, with vaginal cream or jelly. If you are such a woman, the high *success* rate, to put it another way—between 95.5 and 99+ percent—is the rate pertinent for you, not the Hellman-Kistner rates. It is striking that Dr. Hellman repeatedly has used the low 90 percent figure in public statements without explaining it. In doing so, of course, he has, as in other instances related in this book, done a selling job for The Pill, perhaps inadvertently.

Similar distortions exist regarding vaginal foam, which avoids the messiness of the diaphragm, requires no special training or fitting of the user, leaves nothing to remove after intercourse, makes douching wholly unnecessary, is inexpensive to use, and is recognized to be so safe that the Food and Drug Administration allows it to be sold without a prescription. And—as will be discussed—it is highly reliable. Yet Dr. Kistner, in his new book *The Pill: Facts and Fallacies about Today's Oral Contraceptives* (New York City: Delacorte Press, 1969), dismisses vaginal foam (page 26) without noting that it is highly reliable; and in a table listing pregnancy rates (page 32) the foam, oddly, is not mentioned at all. Nor is it mentioned by Dr. Hellman in an article in *Redbook* for April 1969. Dr. Fielding, who prepared a "Complete Guide to Modern Birth Control" for the July 1967 *Ladies' Home Journal,* said that "if used consistently" vaginal foam has a failure rate of "about 1.5 percent." Authorities may differ about that figure, but the efficacy of foam is widely agreed not to be significantly different statistically than that of the diaphragm properly used. The intrauterine devices (IUDs) are believed to be almost as effective as combination versions of The Pill when they stay in place, which is estimated to be 80 percent of the time. But it should be noted that IUDs are not designed for women who have not been pregnant because of pain during insertion and because of the risk of damage to the uterus.

To sum up then, The Pill is not really that much more

"foolproof" than other contraceptive methods. And there are definite dangers involved in using The Pill: A cause-effect relation between The Pill and blood-clotting diseases that can kill and cause permanent disablement has been established; and a long list of other hazards are, in varying degrees, established or suspected and not disproved. But there is no evidence worthy of the name that use of a diaphragm or of spermicidal foam can cause clotting or any other serious disease, or can significantly impair the normal functioning of the body in any way.

For *you*, then, the question—the literally vital question—may be simply, "What price the convenience of The Pill?"

Eighth, someday there may be a means of effective conception control far safer than anything now available—for example, progestogen-only pills implanted under the skin in an artificial rubber material that will diffuse the hormone into the body system at a constant but very low rate; or a vaccination that will make a woman immune to her husband's sperm. In fiscal 1969 alone the National Institute of Child Health and Human Development, one of the National Institutes of Health, let contracts for research and development in contraception for 3.1 million dollars, and the Agency for International Development for 1.5 million dollars; in the current fiscal year the Institute intends to let contracts totaling about 15 million dollars. One can only hope for success. But one must hope at least as urgently that safety will be demonstrated in advance of mass use so that we will not have replays of The Pill story —in which safety was blithely assumed, not established.

Finally, I hope you will read this book with regard to the implications that go beyond The Pill. I refer mainly to a blind, unquestioning faith in technology which amounts to saying that if we have the capacity to make it or build it we ought to; that we then ought to use it, and that the results, of course, will be beneficial. Our experience with DDT and other pesticides raises some questions about these assumptions. So does the neglect of urban rapid transit in favor of an overwhelming reliance on the automobile, with resultant pollution of the atmosphere and a massive toll of death and injury. So does the Supersonic Transport with its threat of sonic booms. So does the construction of nuclear power plants with their threat of thermal pollution. "Since we make so little effort to investigate the effects of social and technological innovations on human life," the distinguished scientist René Dubos said last January in *The New York Times,* "we are practicing—not by intention but irresponsibly—a kind of biological warfare against nature, ourselves, and especially against our descendants."

The Uncontrolled Experiment I

"The oral contraceptives present society with problems unique in the history of human therapeutics. Never will so many people have taken such potent drugs voluntarily over such a protracted period for an objective other than the control of disease."

> —From the report of the Advisory Committee on Obstetrics and Gynecology of the Food and Drug Administration, August 1966.

"A healthy population of women in the child-bearing years, eight million in this country alone, now serve as guinea pigs, where a few carefully monitored subjects would have been sufficient." [1]

> —Dr. Sumner H. Kalman, professor of pharmacology at Stanford University School of Medicine, in *Stanford M.D.*, Fall/Winter 1968–69 issue.

[1] Eight million users in the United States may be as good an estimate as any, but no one really knows for certain how many millions are using oral contraceptives, or how many additional millions have stopped using them. In 1967, for what it is worth, the Population Council estimated the users at 6.5 million in this country and 6.3 million elsewhere.

READ CAREFULLY BEFORE SIGNING

During most of the time that I have been reporting on The Pill the issue was precisely the one suggested by Dr. Kalman —whether millions of women in fact were serving as guinea pigs in a massive, uncontrolled, unscientific experiment. To put it another way, the issue was whether the relative safety of The Pill had been established by careful studies *before* large-scale use was allowed to begin. The answer was that the safety of The Pill had *not* been demonstrated; the reader will find ample documentation of this charge in this book. In the spring of 1967, however, a fundamental change in the nature of the issue occurred with publication of a report by the British Medical Research Council that contained this jolting statement: There "can be no reasonable doubt that some types of thromboembolic disorder are associated with the use of oral contraceptives." This was based on the first solid evidence that in some women The Pill causes blood-clotting diseases that can kill and disable for life. A year later, more complete data caused the FDA to call a meeting with the American manufacturers of The Pill that resulted in a drastic revision of the FDA-approved labeling or prescribing instructions. It was now not only conceded but emphasized that the risk of death or of injury serious enough to require hospitalization from clotting diseases was seven to ten times greater in users of The Pill than in comparable non-users. There are those physicians who question such data on the assumption that reliance is more properly placed in their uncontrolled observations. For these doctors there is, in addition to the approximately 200 pending damage suits brought by victims and their survivors, a new persuader devised by the Nettleship Company of Los Angeles, which administers malpractice insurance programs for 12,000 medical and osteopathic physicians in Southern California and for 6000 osteopathic physicians elsewhere in the nation. On May 14, 1969, John C. Allen, president of the brokerage firm, the second largest of its kind, sent his clients this "claims prevention letter":

Dear Doctor:
    Because of the increasing awareness of potential complications from contraceptive pills, and because we are already handling lawsuits dealing with some of these compli-

cations, we are advising physicians to obtain signed statements from their patients which acknowledge requests for these pills despite awareness of the serious risks involved.

We offer the enclosed form which can be used in most instances.

The enclosed form is reproduced here:

CONTRACEPTIVE DRUGS

Read Carefully Before Signing!

The Prescription for contraceptive drugs on this date and for every refill hereafter is at my request. In making this request, I am aware that such drugs can cause serious reactions and complications, both known and presently unknown.

Date:————————Signature of Patient:————————

"A DIPLOMATIC IMMUNITY"

"In general," Dr. Herbert Ratner said in the Spring 1968 issue of *Child and Family,* "favorable findings of drug-company-subsidized physicians, promoters of The Pill, and naive physicians have been encouraged, widely distributed, scientifically inflated, maximized, and extolled, whereas unfavorable findings have either been ignored, suppressed, rationalized, minimized, or ridiculed." [2] But why?

A key point is that The Pill is a prescription drug. You cannot legally buy it without an authorization—a prescription —from a physician. The physician-patient relationship is built on the presumption that in medical matters the doctor knows best—that he would not prescribe The Pill (or any drug) unless he had good reason to judge that doing so was relatively safe. How would he know that? For one thing, he would take your medical history to find out if you have had a clotting episode or other condition that precludes use of The Pill, and he would examine you for, say, a possible carcinoma of the breast. Advocates of The Pill merchandised the notion that these procedures were sufficient. They were *not.*

[2] A quarterly owned, edited, and published by the National Commission on Human Life Reproduction and Rhythm, Oak Park, Ill.

The most careful and perceptive diagnostician could not, on
the basis of a favorable history and examination, determine if
you were one of those women predisposed to clotting on The
Pill; neither could he detect a latent cancer in the breast. (If,
later on, he were to find a lump, cancer would already be
well along.)

Doctors also leaned heavily on "experts"—those who often
achieve that status simply by espousing "the most popular
and widely held views of the predominant orthodoxy," as
Paul Talalay wrote in *Drugs in Our Society* (Baltimore:
Johns Hopkins Press, 1964). "The history of medicine
abounds with examples of totally illogical treatments . . . because of the powerful influence of an authoritarian orthodoxy," he said. The history of The Pill abounds not only with
illogic but with misstatement of facts—and worse. And that
history abounds, too, with evidence that physicians put their
trust in purported experts blindly, without examining the nature and quality of their evidence.

Take the case of Dr. Joseph W. Goldzieher, chairman of
the Southwest Foundation for Research and Education in San
Antonio, and a consultant to Eli Lilly & Company, maker of
C-Quens, the sequential oral contraceptive. "If the instructions of the physician are followed on taking and how to take
the pills, I can imagine no danger whatsoever," he said on
This Hour Has Seven Days, a television program carried on
February 6, 1966, by the Canadian Broadcasting System. "I
can think of no condition in which these pills would not be
safe to take." Another expert is Dr. Alan F. Guttmacher,
president of Planned Parenthood-World Population and,
among other things, an advisor on family planning to *Consumer Reports.*[3] For years, in pressing for action against the
truly awesome problems of world population growth, he has
nurtured the hope that The Pill was a substantial part of the
answer; therefore, it would be counter-productive to seriously
question its safety. He is responsible in significant measure
for The Pill having acquired what Dr. David B. Clark, a Uni-

---

[3] Published by Consumers Union, which says it "is not beholden in
any way to any commercial interest." But Dr. Guttmacher has evi-
denced a *special* interest in a cause in which The Pill has figured prominently. Such a special interest can be just as productive of bias as a
"commercial interest." Personally, I rate Consumers Union's choice of
family planning consultants such as Dr. Guttmacher "not acceptable,"
and I speak as a member of CU for 33 years.

versity of Kentucky neurologist, has called "a diplomatic immunity" from criticism.

This kind of thing was par for the course: On February 17, 1966, a public relations outfit retained by drug manufacturers sent a handout to news media headlined "ORAL CONTRACEPTIVES NOT CAUSE OF THROMBOEMBOLISMS: DR. GUTTMACHER." The text began, "Fears of thromboembolic involvement in women taking oral contraceptives have no basis in proven medical fact, according to Dr. Alan F. Guttmacher. . . ." The handout was derived from a piece he had written for a throwaway magazine distributed by a drug (not Pill) manufacturer to *general practitioners*. Now that the British studies have established that oral contraceptives *are* a cause of thromboembolisms, however, Dr. Guttmacher's emphasis has undergone a radical shift. "We've never given The Pill a completely clean bill of health," he told C. P. Gilmore, science editor of Metromedia television, for an article published on July 20, 1969, by *The New York Times Magazine*. "It's a powerful drug, and I think one has to be honest and say there is a risk with any powerful drug."

In addition to the experts, the Food and Drug Administration played a role in fostering the faith much of the medical profession had in the safety of The Pill. Doctors assumed that it would not have been admitted to the market had its safety not been demonstrated in advance to the FDA. But for the most part they were not even faintly aware of the gross ineptitude that prevailed in the FDA. For years, for example, the agency authorized conflicting labeling for identical formulations. Thus when norethindrone plus mestranol was sold as Norinyl, there appeared under "contraindications," the most urgent portion of the labeling, the admonishment to discontinue the product in patients with a history of psychic depression "if depression recurs to a marked degree." When the same formulation was sold as Ortho-Novum, however, nothing at all about psychic depression appeared in the contraindications; instead there appeared in the mild "precautions" section only a suggestion that patients with a history of depression "be carefully observed." And doctors who turned to the Committee on Human Reproduction of the American Medical Association, whose report on "The Control of Fertility" was published on October 25, 1965, in the *Journal* of the AMA, were cryptically advised, "Safety must always be demonstrated [to the FDA] before a new drug application [for marketing] can be made. . . ." [4]

In our governmental system of checks and balances the Congress is supposed to oversee the performance of the Executive Branch. Although this function is incredibly neglected, it actually worked, to some extent and for a time, in the case of The Pill. For two and one half years the Senate Subcommittee on Executive Reorganization, headed by then Senator Hubert H. Humphrey, conducted an inquiry into the FDA that reached its handling of the oral contraceptives. But the inquiry was aborted in 1964 when Humphrey became the Democratic candidate for vice president.

The Founding Fathers, in the First Amendment, guaranteed freedom of the press. Here, too, there were grave failures of commission and omission. For example, Julius N. Cahn, the dedicated one-man professional staff of the Humphrey Subcommittee, obtained from FDA files a shocking internal document prepared in May 1960 by Dr. William D. Kessenich, who was then director of the Bureau of Medicine. The paper notified the late Commissioner George P. Larrick that the New Drug Branch of the Bureau had "concluded that the evidence establishes the safety of Enovid tablets [Enovid, a product of G. D. Searle, & Co., Inc., was the pioneer oral contraceptive] for use in conception control. . . ." The nature and quality of "the evidence" was hidden from the press, medical profession, and public by policies of rigid secrecy which the FDA had used to protect itself from critical examination about large-scale blunders, such as the release of numerous prescription drugs that later had to be recalled from the market as unsafe. And so in the absence of disclosure about what "the evidence" was, the general assumption was that the FDA was observing a high standard of safety of the kind laid down in August 1961 in the *American Journal of Obstetrics and Gynecology* by four members of the Harvard Medical School faculty: "No method of pregnancy spacing,

---

[4] In a letter to me immediately after the report was issued, Dr. Louis Lasagna of the Johns Hopkins School of Medicine said that "the article, in its concern for the benefits [of population control] to be obtained from effective contraception, neglects what I consider to be all too definite warning signals on the horizon in regard to the ability of the oral contraceptives to cause vascular catastrophe. I admit that I am probably in the minority in feeling so concerned and in feeling so impressed by the available evidence, but the majority is often wrong, as you know."

even though highly effective, is justifiable if it endangers life or health," they said. Strengthening the assumption was the publicity given the tests of Enovid in significant numbers of women in Puerto Rico, Haiti, and California; but these tests were for efficacy.

Early in 1963 the Humphrey Subcommittee published the Kessenich document, which was the foundation for the FDA decision three years earlier to let Enovid be marketed as a contraceptive (it had been sold since 1957 for therapeutic purposes such as endometriosis and hypermenorrhea). The paper disclosed that the "entire series of clinical cases"—the foundation for the conclusion of safety—included a mere 132 women who had received Enovid *continuously* for a year or more. Half—66—had taken the tablets for 12 to 21 *consecutive* menstrual cycles; half had taken them for 24 to a maximum of 38 *consecutive* cycles. "Continuously" and "consecutive" are the operative words, because brief or occasional ingestion of powerful chemicals is not an adequate test of safety for a human being who, so far as anyone knew, might be taking The Pill for as long as three decades—the childbearing age span from 15 to 44. But though the Enovid was administered "continuously," the inadequacy of the sample was a scandal.

If there are 8 million American women on The Pill, the number destined to suffer a fatal, causally related clotting episode in 1969 will exceed by more than 100 the number of women in the test sample. Yet when the figures were disclosed in the printed hearings of the Humphrey Subcommittee they got almost no attention in the press or anywhere else. And so, perhaps, it was not too surprising that there was no mention of them two and one half years later in the guide to conception control published in the *Journal* of the AMA by its Committee on Human Reproduction. The committee chairman, Dr. Raymond T. Holden, a Washington obstetrician, acknowledged in an interview that neither he nor, so far as he was aware, the seven members of the committee had heard of the figures in the Kessenich document. Of course, Dr. Holden said, 132 women were "not enough" for presuming safety in long-term use by millions of women.

In addition to relying on experts, the AMA, the FDA, Congress, and the news media, physicians were influenced by the drumfire of publicity and promotion from manufacturers of The Pill. This element should not be underestimated. Although it is widely known that the drug industry is consistently the nation's most profitable, it is not generally grasped that this profitability is tied to an expenditure for promotion and advertising of $4500 per physician per year, according to an estimate in 1968 of the Prescription Drug Task Force of the Department of Health, Education, and Welfare. This kind of money talks—and talks much more loudly than an occasional cautionary article in a medical or scientific journal (usually a British one, in the initial years of oral contraception). You can readily understand my point from your own experience with television. Repeatedly you have seen commercials for the "whitener" toothpaste that is supposed to give your mouth "sex appeal." Lacking a commercial sponsor, the message of the Council on Dental Therapeutics of the American Dental Association gets through to very few people, the message being that "whitener" toothpastes may be excessively abrasive and possibly harmful to the one over-35 adult in four whose gums have started to recede and expose the relatively soft dentum.

And so we will look at some of the activities of producers of The Pill. The principal one is G. D. Searle & Company, Incorporated, of Chicago. This is a profitable enterprise, thanks in substantial part to The Pill—various versions of Enovid and Ovulen-21. In 1968, for example, net earnings *after* taxes were $27,370,000 on sales of $147,700,000, or more than 18 percent; in 1964, net earnings after taxes were $12,100,000, or 28.2 percent of sales of $42,900,000. It should be borne in mind that a more significant figure is a rate of return on net worth, or investment. This is the standard economic measure, the one that informs investors so that they can compare the premiums which their risk dollars can earn. Searle's rate of return under this measure was 27.9 percent in 1968 and 38.9 percent in 1964. (The intervening years were comparably bountiful.)

In December 1967 Searle published an advertisement for Ovulen-21 in the *Journal* of the American Medical Association and in a magazine for obstetricians and gynecologists. At the time the official, FDA-authorized labeling said that a cause-effect relation with blood clotting and damage to the nervous tissue of the eyes "has been *neither established nor disproved*" [emphasis supplied]. This balanced statement, later strengthened to acknowledge a causal association, had been approved in June 1967 to take effect in advertising of all brands of The Pill on October 1 of that year. Needless to say, Searle was fully aware of this, having agreed to it in negotiations with the FDA and having included it in the brochure of every package it was sending to pharmacists. Searle also well knew, of course, that since 1962, the Kefauver-Harris Amendments to the Food, Drug, and Cosmetic Act had required that "all descriptive matter" for prescription drugs carry "a true statement . . . in brief summary" of the contraindications, warnings, precautions, and side effects in the official labeling. Finally, it may be assumed that Searle was sophisticated enough to realize that the more it played down safety considerations, the less the inhibition on physicians to prescribe the company's products.

With all of these considerations in mind, let us return to the Ovulen-21 ad published five months after the neither-proved-nor-disproved statement was approved and two months after its use was required. Instead of using this language, the ad relied instead on the original labeling which, in a weak, unbalanced statement that did not admit a causal relation had not been disproved, said merely that "a cause and effect relationship has not been established."

A principal mechanism used by the FDA to deal with advertising violations is the corrective letter, the inspiration of Dr. Robert S. McCleery, a brilliant, dedicated public servant who had been head of the FDA's Medical Advertising Branch. Such a letter enables quick correction of a misleading ad with a communication mailed individually to each physician. The agency has "clout" to compel a reluctant manufacturer to go along—the power and willingness of the FDA, if it comes to that, to seize interstate shipments of the misadvertised product. In a "Dear Doctor" letter dated January 26, 1968, Searle contritely admitted that the Ovulen-21 ads had departed from the "neither established nor disproved" labeling "in several respects" and that it had relied on the earlier labeling which "did not accurately represent the present status of opinion concerning the possible danger of side effects." [5] The letter, signed by Herbert Helling, Searle's liaison with FDA, went on to say:

[5] The very first corrective letter, dated February 1, 1967, was sent by the Ortho Pharmaceutical Corporation to apologize to the medical profession for an ad for Ortho-Novum SQ. Later, similar apologies were sent by Mead Johnson Laboratories for an ad for Oracon and by Syntex Laboratories for ads for Norquen and Norinyl-1. These letters are reproduced in Appendix A.

The FDA regards the advertisements as potentially misleading because they omitted this important change [to the
newer labeling] which emphasizes the possibility of these
serious hazards.

Further, the advertisements failed to include the following side effects which, although causation has not been established, have been reported in users of oral contraceptives: anovulation post treatment, premenstrual-like syndrome, changes in libido, changes in appetite, cystitis-like
syndrome, backache, nervousness, dizziness, fatigue, headache, hirsutism.

We have modified our advertising to reflect these
changes.

There was another and more subtle area than advertising
about which doctors were misled. This concerned a quite natural assumption that such fatal reactions as were reported in
women on The Pill were conscientiously and routinely investigated by the manufacturers. That this was by no means always true was disclosed by Dr. Schuyler G. Kohl, who was
retained as a special consultant by the Advisory Committee
on Obstetrics and Gynecology for its report of August 1966
to the Food and Drug Administration. In February and
March of 1966 Dr. Kohl, professor of obstetrics and gynecology at the State University of New York in Brooklyn, visited
the seven companies that were then making The Pill. In a review of his findings, published as an appendix to the committee report, Dr. Kohl said he had found the company physicians and scientists "truly concerned about the safety of the
medications their firms produce." He also found these men to
be aware of "shortcomings" in their methods of surveillance
of trouble in women on The Pill, meaning, of course, that the
incidence was understated. Without naming any names, Dr.
Kohl said:

The "medical departments" of the manufacturers are
quite variable. Some are very sophisticated in approach
and personnel, and one occupies a "basement office" and is
quite restricted in personnel and outlook. . . .

It was anticipated, prior to the visits, that there would be
a degree of uniformity in the records and investigations of
reported deaths. The variability was marked and so was

the degree of responsibility and involvement. Some of the investigations of deaths were associated with repeated visits and telephone calls to physicians whose patients had died. Other investigations were quite cursory and *reflected considerable concern over the company's image with the physician. "He cannot be irritated—it's bad for our business relationships"* [emphasis supplied].

Now that we have looked briefly at circumstances that contributed to a regrettable lack of wariness about The Pill in the medical profession, it is time to examine the nature and origins of some of the pressures that patients came to apply on doctors.

IMPRUDENCE AND THE PILL

There is in the United States a myth, one that has been most tenacious, that science is all silver lining and no cloud. This myth usually finds expression in such notions as that if it's new it must be better, and that there will be, if there isn't already, a pill for every ill. Not that such notions are original with Americans. Even the ancient Hippocrates, in *On Wounds of the Head, I,* mocked those who "praise what seems outlandish before they know whether it is good, rather than the customary which they already know to be good; the bizzare rather than the obvious." In 1896 Elihu Thomson found that X-rays injured body tissues; in 1927 Hermann J. Muller, the geneticist who ultimately was awarded a Nobel Prize, reported that X-rays cause mutations of the genes. Yet in 1923 there spread across the United States and Canada a business employing beauticians to remove unwanted hair with X-ray treatments—an enterprise rooted in a faith that such a stunning symbol of scientific achievement as X-rays had to be benign. The business flourished for six years. The consequences included thousands of cases of X-ray burns, cancer, and even death. Now the point is not that X-rays were not a great step forward for mankind, because they were. The point is that we did not display a mature and respectful wisdom about how to use X-rays that was on a par with our innovative technology. And this is my point about The Pill. It is a magnificent achievement of the biological sciences; but it was outlandish that, as Dr. Herbert Ratner has said, "the real users of The Pill, the middle and upper classes of the U.S.,

were seduced away from well established and safe means of
birth control"—from, in Hippocrates' phrase, "the customary
which they already know to be good." It was unwise, it was
bizarre, to have allowed this seduction to have occurred,
whereas it was not bizarre for The Pill to have been seized
upon, as the British medical magazine *Lancet* has said, "in
overcrowded lands, where starvation for the many is a more
serious and immediate threat than uncertainty about future ill
health in a few. . . ." As in the case of X-rays, there was in
the worshipful attitude with which the middle and upper
classes approach technology, the mental set that allowed
promoters and popularizers to accomplish the seduction with
remarkably little resistance. Women and men alike wanted to
believe in the safety of The Pill, with its convenience ("No
more greasy kid stuff," a friend of mine said), its efficacy, its
contribution to a new sexual freedom. They believed what
they wanted to believe.

But they surely were helped along. One of the helpers was
Dr. Robert A. Wilson, a Brooklyn, New York, gynecologist
who preached that The Pill can make women youthful, sexy
and, in the words of the title of his popular book, *Feminine
Forever*. In the first seven months after its publication in January 1966 the book sold 100,000 copies. Dr. Wilson was syn-
dicated by newspapers, excerpted by *Look* and *Vogue*, made
tantalizing by *Time*. With doses of synthetic estrogen, which
the ovaries stop producing in the middle years, and of a synthetic progestogen, he said he could make sex more enjoyable
"regardless of age," and told of his "crash program" to pre-
pare a 72-year-old English woman for her wedding night.

Although he is a leading proponent of The Pill, Dr. Robert
W. Kistner of Harvard says he is "suspicious (to put it
mildly) about the fantastic claims of the 'feminine forever'
school." On March 19, 1966, writing in the *New Republic*,
James Ridgeway and Nancy Sommers reported that the Wilson Research Foundation, headed by Dr. Wilson, had received, in 1964, $17,000 from the Searle Foundation, which
was created by the Searles of G. D. Searle & Company;
$8700 from Ayerst Laboratories, and $5600 from the Upjohn Company. In his writings Dr. Wilson claimed that the
menopause could be prevented with the use of birth control
pills. When he shunned mention of Searle's Enovid, he spoke
of norethynodrel, a synthetic progestogen found only in Enovid. He told George Lardner, Jr., of the *Washington Post*

that he personally does not prescribe The Pill, favoring instead prescribing "conjugated estrogens" supplemented by a progestogen. "Conjugated estrogens" are a speciality of Ayerst Laboratories; the progestogen he named, medroxy-progesterone acetate, is made by Upjohn. The Searle firm was Dr. Wilson's research sponsor. In November 1966 the Food and Drug Administration notified the company that Dr. Wilson had "publicized the use of Enovid in lay publications, stating that it is effective in preventing symptoms of the menopause. Our investigational drug regulations provide that neither the sponsor nor anyone on its behalf may disseminate promotional material claiming that the drug has been shown to be effective for the conditions for which it is being investigated. Dr. Wilson has disseminated such information. He is therefore unacceptable as an investigator for 'Enovid in the Menopause.' "

Starting in 1963, the Searle firm made annual grants, in unspecified amounts, to Dr. J. Ernest Ayre, medical and scientific director of the National Cancer Cytology Center of New York and Miami. The Center put out a press release for use on June 29, 1966, with this headline: " 'THE PILL' FOUND SAFE FOR USE BY PATIENTS WITH EARLY CERVICAL CANCER—*Research by Cytology Center Will Ease Fears of Millions Who Take Oral Contraceptives*"

The press release was used by newspapers including the *Evening Star* in Washington. It announced the results of a "daring three-year study of the influence of the pioneer birth control pill," which further on was clearly identified as Enovid, on women "predisposed to cancer of the cervix." Adding powerfully to the credibility of the release was the information that the results were being published in *Obstetrics and Gynecology,* the official journal of the American College of Obstetricians and Gynecologists. The study "should remove many of the doubts of those who prescribe and those who take oral contraceptives," the release said. Dr. Ayre hawked his message to the Associated Press, which, on May 10, 1967, sent over its wires an interview in which Dr. Ayre made the claim that studies showed Enovid will not cause, and may inhibit, cervical cancer. The simple fact, however, is that Dr. Ayre's study should have removed none of the doubts which he had cited. The reasons are summed up by the FDA's Advisory Committee on Obstetrics and Gynecology in its 1966 report. The committee, drawing on a review of all available data on cervical cancer by a Task Force on Carcinogenic Potential headed by Dr. Roger B. Scott, professor of obstetrics and gynecology at Western Reserve University in Cleveland, Ohio, said, "It is to be emphasized that all known human carcinogens require a latent period of approximately one decade. Hence any valid conclusion must await accurate data on a much larger group of women [than had been carefully studied by Dr. Ayre or anyone else] studied for at least ten years. Furthermore, there is not sufficient evidence to support the contention that contraceptive pills may protect against the development of carcinoma of the cervix."

In addition to his work with the Cytology Center, Dr. Ayre was medical consultant to the Rand Development Corporation of Cleveland (not to be confused with the RAND Corporation of Santa Monica, California) which, with the indispensable aid of cover stories in the December 1966 and January 1967 issues of *Pageant* magazine, was promoting a purported cancer vaccine for terminal victims. The FDA petitioned for an injunction to prevent further manufacture and distribution of the vaccine. If the laboratory in which it had been produced had been "a butcher shop, it would have been closed up by the health authorities," the late United States Attorney Merle M. McCurdy told District Judge James C. Connell in a hearing held on Rand Development's objections to the government's petition. Yet Dr. Ayre testified that he administered the vaccine—which was promoted for *terminal* cancer victims—to women whose cervical tissue had been diagnosed as *pre-cancerous*. The vaccine was untested and some of it, the government brought out, was contaminated; some may even have contained a carcinogen known as benzidine. Dr. Ayre took 150 to 200 vials from Ohio to physicians in other states and even to the Dominican Republic. The law concerning drugs that are legally in investigational or experimental status prohibits removal of the vials of the vaccine from Ohio and testing outside the boundaries of that state. Dr. Ayre knew, the judge said, that every vial administered outside of Ohio was administered in violation of the law. Dr. Ayre's explanation understandably left the judge incredulous: "He said he administered vaccine to patients for psychological purposes . . . to make them feel good." I called all of this to the attention of G. D. Searle & Company and asked whether the grant to Dr. Ayre would be renewed later in 1967. It was. On December 13, 1968, a Federal grand jury in Cleveland indicted Rand Development and its president, H. James Rand, on three counts of mail fraud and three of securities fraud. They have pleaded innocent.

Claude Bernard, the great French physiologist, said a century ago that "true science teaches us to doubt and in ignorance to refrain." Drs. Ayre and Wilson, financially aided by a company which exists to make money and which has admitted to physicians that it advertised one of its Pills in ways that overstated the evidence of safety, tried to teach the women of America *not* to doubt and in ignorance *not* to refrain from ingesting potent chemicals 20 days a month. As Dr. Herbert Ratner said in *Child and Family* for Summer 1968, "women make superb guinea pigs—they don't cost anything, feed themselves, clean their own 'cages,' pay for their own Pills and remunerate the clinical observer," all contrary to the letter and spirit of the requirement of the Food, Drug, and Cosmetic Act of 1938 that safety be demonstrated *before a drug goes on the market.*

The process by which women who were told over and over that The Pill was SAFE, and by which millions of them were persuaded, was impeded by few if any outcries in news media from leaders of medicine, some of whom were meanwhile anguishing in private. The following is an example of the conflict between the "persuaders" and those who seriously questioned the safety of The Pill:

On October 15, 1965, the Searle firm undertook a highly unusual campaign against my book, *The Therapeutic Nightmare.* It contained a chapter factually summarizing the reasons why responsible scientists were concerned whether the safety of The Pill had been established. The company retaliated by distributing an eight-page "Fact Sheet" to book-review editors and book reviewers all over the country. The headline was "SEARLE SEEKS TO AVOID PUBLIC 'PANIC' ON ORAL CONTRACEPTIVES BY ALERTING BOOK REVIEWERS TO 'MISINFORMATION' IN MINTZ BOOK." The text said there was a "danger that if certain statements from the book are given wide circulation without amplifying or qualifying data, literally *millions* of American women may be thrown into panic regarding the safety of *all* oral contraceptives." The book had raised questions about whether The Pill could cause clotting; the "Fact Sheet" tried to show that no basis existed for raising such questions and that I therefore was some kind of cheap sensationalist; yet today there is labeling on Searle's Pills in which the FDA and the company agree that The Pill multiplies the risk of fatal and serious clotting seven to ten times.

Promotions such as Dr. Wilson's and Dr. Ayre's were, of course, only a small part of the avalanche of pro-Pill pressures exerted on women to use The Pill. If you picked up the Helen Gurley Brown book *Sex and the Office* (New York City: Bernard Geis Associates, 1964), you would be advised in the chapter on management of an affair during the lunch hour: "If you use pills, so much the easier." If you picked up *McCall's* for May 1967 you would read that Jeanine Deckers, the former Singing Nun, had composed "La Pilule d'Or" ("The Golden Pill"); in her fresh, beautiful voice "she was singing a hymn of praise to God for inspiring mankind to invent the birth-control pill." If you went to the movies you might see *Prudence and the Pill,* a 20th Century-Fox production described by a *New York Times* reviewer as "a nauseating little sex comedy in which somebody is always substituting a vitamin or an aspirin for somebody else's oral contraceptive until everyone gets confused or pregnant." If you read *Life* for July 3, 1964, to find out what Dr. Joseph F. Sadusk, Jr., the top doctor in the Food and Drug Administration, had to say, you would be given reassurance: "We are not taking a dogmatic attitude that oral contraceptives are absolutely safe—and we do intend to review the evidence immediately. But the indications so far are that they are safe, when given under the supervision of a doctor. . . . We are not worried. But we're going to watch it."

It would have been better to watch Dr. Sadusk. After two years of decision-making that repeatedly favored the drug producers over the drug consumers, he left the agency and after a pause became vice president of Parke-Davis & Co. Its products include Norlestrin, an oral contraceptive. Even more reassuring than Dr. Sadusk was Gregory Pincus, a pioneer in the development of The Pill. In the *Ladies' Home Journal* for June 1963 he recited a long list of "ills," including, preposterously, "a tendency to blood clotting," that one person or another had attributed to the drugs. "When subjected to careful scrutiny, all of these conditions have been found to be unrelated to the use of the contraceptives," he said. Five years later, Robert A. Liston, author of *What You Should Know about Pills,* was, if you can believe it, even more sure of their safety. He said that for years women had been taking The Pill "with no ill effects." [6]

The whole milieu was appropriate to a stampede. And there was one to the doctors' offices. Once in the corral the women did not lack for reading matter; pamphlets intended to prevent second thoughts were thoughtfully provided by the manufacturers. These stimulated a desire for one or another brand of The Pill even before the physician who was acting as a salesman had taken a patient's medical history or examined her. In dealing with such pamphlets it will be sufficient to cite "A Word to the Wives," a slick propaganda job done by Ortho Pharmaceutical Corporation in October 1965. "Ortho-Novum will not reduce your future ability to have a baby," the brochure said. This flat statement is open to severe challenge, as is discussed later in this book; and the FDA labeling for Ortho-Novum said that "the possible effects on organs of the body such as the pituitary gland, *ovaries,* adrenal glands and uterus must await observations from continuing studies" [emphasis supplied]. "Ortho-Novum Tablets have been proven safe," the pamphlet said. That statement was incorrect. So was another: "Ortho-Novum does not interfere with your state of well-being." The state of well-being of a good many users was interfered with. Let it be said, however, that for physicians with a more balanced attitude toward The Pill, Ortho had a more balanced pamphlet, which is not surprising because the company is a conception control conglomerate: it makes not only The Pill, but also Delfen Vaginal Foam (which, along with the Emko brand, is listed by the Medical Committee of the Planned Parenthood Federation of America), vaginal creams and jellies (both those intended for use with diaphragms and the spermicidal forms intended for use without them), diaphragms, and IUDs. The pamphlet, "A Woman's Guide to the Methods of Postponing or Preventing Pregnancy," was, in stark contrast to "A Word to the Wives," at least an attempt to put the var-

---

[6] In the foreword to *The Pill: Facts and Fallacies about Today's Oral Contraceptives,* Dr. Robert W. Kistner says, "To assist me in the conversion of mysterious medical terminology to acceptable language, I have utilized the talents of a gifted writer, Robert A. Liston."

ious techniques in some perspective.[7] But by and large the
Pill-pushing pamphlets had a simple, seductive theme: The
way for you to harmonize your life is to hormonize it. Necessarily the sales potential in such a proposition would have
been weakened by an emphasis on, or even a mention of,
warnings and side effects.[8]

What does it all add up to—the uncritical beginnings, the
exuberant experts, the "diplomatic immunity" from criticism,
the failures of a government agency with a mission to protect
the public health, the AMA committee of experts that had
not heard of the miniscule test sample of 132 women even
though it had been disclosed in the printed hearings of a
congressional subcommittee, the advertisements that could
mislead the doctor and injure or possibly kill the helpless patient, the sloppy company records on Pill victims, and the ex-
ploitation of women who trusted the experts, the leaders of
medicine, and the FDA by books, song, movie, articles, pamphlets?

The sum of elements such as these is a potential for disas-
ter. This applies not only to The Pill, but to nuclear power,
pesticides, and other products of technology that are not han-
dled judiciously. I wish I could say I am satisfied that we will
not have more uncontrolled mass experiments such as that
with The Pill, but I am not. There are strong forces whose
thrust is not to let the lessons of The Pill be instructive but to
put them out of mind; to talk about the marvels of what is
coming rather than the troubles of what is already here; to
forget the past rather than to learn from it.

The title of C. P. Gilmore's article in *The New York
Times Magazine* for July 20, 1969, was "Something Better
Than the Pill?" In it Dr. Louis M. Hellman, the leading out-

---

[7] I am speaking of versions which dropped from page 3 this griev-
ously and dangerously misleading paragraph in the edition dated May
1967: "None of the methods mentioned in this book is harmful to a
woman in normal health. None of them will reduce her ability to have
a child, if she wants one, in the future." The edition dated May 1968
substituted, "Your doctor is the best source of information regarding
safety. He will not prescribe a method unless he feels it will be safe for
you, his patient."

[8] In September 1967 the FDA finally cracked down on this kind of
double standard applied at the point of sale. The agency ruled that
instruction booklets, as well as "ostensibly educational films and au-
dio-visual materials" that discuss safety and efficacy must list adverse
information and warnings fully and in language understandable to the
patient.

side consultant to the government of the United States on contraception, said, "If there *is* going to be cancer, then it would take at least ten years to show up so we could recognize it. That would be 1972 at the earliest, probably five years later. And I think we'll be well away from the present Pills by then."

How reassuring.

Blood Clotting II

A blood clot forms in an inflamed vein in the leg or pelvis. A piece breaks away and travels to, and blocks, the lung artery or a blood vessel in the brain. The consequences of these painful conditions—respectively, thrombophlebitis, pulmonary embolism and stroke—include death, lifelong disability, paralysis, eye damage, a stay in the hospital followed by partial or full recovery, or, for the most fortunate, injury not serious enough to require hospitalization or to leave residual effects. Like heart attacks—which the available sound evidence indicates to be rarely if ever causally related to The Pill—these blood-clotting diseases occur spontaneously, that is, without known cause. (They occur, as well, because of identifiable causes such as surgery.) Until the time came when there were well-controlled scientific studies to determine if The Pill was or was not a cause of clotting, randomly reported personal experiences had to be treated with great wariness. They might properly have aroused suspicion and demands for scientific studies; and that is exactly what happened when some practicing physicians began to encounter previously healthy young women who had suffered lung clots, which were the primary initial concern, and strokes. The medical reaction was especially strong in Britain, where doctors are more likely to fire off a letter to a medical journal when they have something to say.

Two points troubled them: Such cases had been very rare, and the ones they now were getting had been on The Pill. In September 1965, for example, a British pathologist performed an inquest on a woman of 22 who had been taking The Pill "since the beginning of the summer" and who suffered a lung clot. "I have never seen a similar case . . . and I have seen many unexpected deaths in young people," the pathologist said at the inquest. "My own feeling is that the association [with use of The Pill] is just too much to be a

38

coincidence." At almost the same time, in the *British Medical Journal*, Dr. Geoffrey Rivett expressed concern even though he had between 50 and 100 women on The Pill who had *not* had a clotting episode. "But such figures prove nothing," he said, and ". . . it would be a great help if an authoritative body would carry out a prospective trial" [in which women would be assigned at random to a group that would be started on The Pill, or to control groups on conventional contraception or no contraception at all].

I am going to present three specific cases here not because they "prove" a cause-effect link with The Pill, which they do not, but because the human element should not be buried amidst the facts and arguments.

CASE A

In December 1965 I wrote for the *Washington Post* a detailed analysis of the evidence up to that time about the scientific quality of the testing done to establish whether The Pill might seriously endanger women who used it. The story was distributed to client papers of the *Los Angeles Times/Washington Post News Service* and thus attracted attention around the country. In Louisville, Kentucky, the *Courier-Journal,* after printing the article, reported that Dr. Peggy Howard had called it "irresponsible" and that Mrs. William R. Keys, Jr., executive director of the Planned Parenthood Clinic and Family Relations Center, had called it "disgusting." In addition, Dr. Douglas M. Haynes, professor and chairman of the Department of Obstetrics and Gynecology at the University of Louisville School of Medicine, said, "Studies made to date have shown that *no harmful effects* have resulted from the use of The Pill . . ." [emphasis supplied].

But I know of no physician who was more outraged at finding a journalistic poacher in the preserves of medicine than Dr. Glenn A. Gryte of Boulder, Colorado. After reading my December article in the *Denver Post* he sent me a letter in which he termed the story "an example of the excesses permitted by 'freedom of the press.' " The experts on whom he relies, he told me, are men such as Gregory Pincus and Dr. John Rock, codiscoverers of The Pill, and not on the critics whom I had cited (along with the advocates). One of the critics was Dr. Louis Lasagna, an associate professor of medi-

cine and associate professor of pharmacology and experimental therapeutics at Johns Hopkins University Medical School,
and a consultant to the National Institutes of Health. "Lasagna?" Dr. Gryte said. "My wife cooks it for supper."

Two years later, in March 1968, I had another letter from
Boulder. This one was from a senior at the University of Colorado Law School who told me he had read my article, "The
Golden Pill," in the March 2 *New Republic*. He said, "Last
week my sister died of a blood clot which blocked the left
internal carotid artery. She was twenty-one, had been taking
The Pill for one and one half months and leaves a four-
month-old son." Inquiry established that the girl had not
been a patient of Dr. Gryte.

CASE B

The *New Republic* article mentioned in Case A elicited
several condemnatory letters from doctors, medical students,
and sociologists. One of the protestors was Clark Hinderleider, medical student and research associate in cardiovascu-
lar physiology-surgery at the University of Southern California in Los Angeles. Along with the others, he thought it out-
rageous that a mere *reporter* could venture into a field in
which "pronouncements by medical doctors and authorities
most concerned have been reasoned, cautious and calm." As
an example of such a pronouncement, he said that I had
failed to take into account "species specificity as well as individual genetic variation" which together warrant the conclusion that "the pills are absolutely safe—just some women are
not." Toward the end of his letter Hinderleider injected "a
personal note"—a complaint that I was engendering a response in patients that was "excited and not rational." I had,
he said, engaged in "sensationalism" that was "a disservice to
the women involved as well as to medical and allied sciences
trying to investigate in an orderly and rational manner the
effects of the oral contraceptives."

Not everyone agreed that the article was "a disservice."
One such was a woman in Halifax, Nova Scotia, who on
May 25, 1968—four days before Hinderleider went to his
typewriter—said in a letter to the *New Republic* that was for-
warded to me but not printed:

On March 22, 1968, I suffered an attack of thromboembolism which caused a blood clot to travel from my leg to my left lung. The attack was not so severe that I would even have called the doctor if I hadn't, shortly before, read "The Golden Pill." I realized that my symptoms (congestion and pain in the left side of my chest) were described in the article, and that I, who had been on The Pill for three years and who was in the age range of persons who have suffered such attacks, might be having one.[1] I had never had any doubt about the strength of my heart and lungs, so the attack was completely unexpected. Before reading Mintz's article, I would never have suspected that such an attack was possible—I had never had any history of circulatory troubles.

In summary, I'm not sure I would have called the doctor in time and been taken to the emergency section of the local hospital and treated with intravenous doses of heparin [an anti-coagulant] if Mr. Mintz's article had not informed me. Two months later, I am still suffering with phlebitis, but hope that eventually I'll recover from the effects of taking The Pill.

CASE C

The following letter, written to the author on March 21, 1967, was from a woman in Bethesda, Maryland, who had read *The Therapeutic Nightmare* and was especially interested by the chapter on oral contraceptives:

This subject is close to my heart, having, by the Grace of God, survived a thromboembolism after taking oral contraceptives (Ortho-Novum) for two months. I feel certain that my experience was not as rare as one is led to believe from reading newspaper reports, magazine articles, and medical journals (which I perused yesterday at the National Library of Medicine in Bethesda), the majority of which seem to give The Pill a full green light and clean bill of health, no strings attached. I have talked to only one

[1] Dr. N. E. Herrera, of Danbury Hospital in Connecticut, has estimated that in a woman on The Pill who develops coughing, chest pain, fatigue, palpitation, anxiety, or wheezing, the chance that she has suffered a lung clot is 40 percent or larger. The estimate is in a paper prepared for a meeting last year of the College of American Pathologists.

doctor who has been willing to share his doubts on The Pill's safety with me. Certainly the estimated six million American women who are taking oral contraceptives deserve to know more about the risks involved, but how are they to get this information when the ill effects are, I suspect, grossly underreported by doctors, hospitals, and the F.D.A.?

The Pill was prescribed to me, a healthy 44-year-old mother of four sons, the eldest 20, the youngest 11, in July 1965. My obstetrician considered me to be a "good risk," having known me for fourteen years, and delivered without complication my two youngest children. I have enjoyed near perfect health all my life. Just over two months later I developed a serious case of pleurisy, unaccompanied by other symptoms of fever, cold or cough. Five days later, feeling continually exhausted and suffering from excruciating pain in my lower rib area, I went to a general practitioner. After an exhaustive examination, including X-rays, the doctor tried to get a bed for me at George Washington Hospital, but none was available until the next day. He suspected a blood clot, due possibly to the fact that I had had a bad fall several weeks before on the tennis court, and sprained a foot. I returned home with "codeine pills" and kept in touch off and on throughout the day with the doctor. The excruciating pain increased until ten o'clock that night when I experienced dagger-like, massive pains throughout my chest, [and found myself] screaming "I'm dying." A half-hour later, at George Washington Hospital, a dose of heparin alleviated the condition. I spent two weeks in the hospital, and after seven weeks was taken off all medication and declared cured. I have suffered no permanent ill effects from this experience, but my doctor suggested that I not take The Pill again.

My obstetrician, who had originally prescribed oral contraceptives, had, in the meantime, died of a heart attack. The general practitioner (whom I credit with saving my life) has never admitted to the possibility of a causal relationship between the use of Ortho-Novum and the thrombosis, saying it could just have easily been caused by my fall. The next obstetrician I went to, when told of my experience and asked if he didn't have many women on The Pill suffering from similar experiences, would not commit himself, answering merely, "The strangest things happen to people." However, in the hospital when interns and residents interviewed me, the first question was always, "Have you been taking The Pill?" and "For how long?" An eminent chest specialist who was called in to perform a thoracentesis, [a procedure for removal of fluids from the chest cavity] was the only doctor I encountered who was willing to discuss any adverse effects The Pill might have. He was frank in saying that he had seen more women with my trouble in the last few months than he had before in years of practice. He felt that despite reports of sufficient testing, the way Puerto Rican women reacted to oral contraceptives would be quite different from the way American women would react, with an entirely different diet, climate, and way of life.

Since my case was not fatal, neither my husband nor myself has been able to ascertain whether it was reported to any authority such as the FDA.

Last summer, in my own family, my 35-year-old sister, having taken oral contraceptives for about two months, had a severe thrombophlebitis which incapacitated her for several months. She reported to me that her gynecologist would not admit to the possibility of any causal relationship between taking The Pill and her illness.

I would be interested in knowing whether, as a result of your book, you have had letters reporting experiences such as I had. Your article in the Sunday *Washington Post* a little more than a year ago was just about the only article I have seen in the newspapers raising any doubts about The Pill's safety. Having just read that in 1966 it has been estimated that approximately 10 million women throughout the world were taking The Pill (of these, 6 million Americans), it distresses me that some of them should have to suffer what my sister and I did because of not being warned of the potential harmful effects.

MEDICAL CAMOUFLAGE

As noted earlier, blood clotting in the legs, pelvis, lungs, and brain occurs without known cause. This provided a kind of medical camouflage for clotting caused by The Pill. A lack of reliable statistics even for fatal episodes helped to make the camouflage effective. Also enhancing the "cover story" for clotting was the claim that The Pill induces a "natural" and "physiologic" method of contraception. If you buy this idea, which a lot of women did because they understandably preferred being "natural" to being "unnatural," you can quite easily build on it to accept another proposition—that clotting in users must be "natural" and not caused by the drugs.

The leading proponent of this sort of argument is Dr. John Rock, who made it in, among other places, his book *The Time Has Come: A Catholic Doctor's Proposals to End the Battle over Birth Control* (New York City: Alfred A. Knopf, Inc., 1963). The claim has another side to it. In addition to being a codiscoverer of The Pill, Dr. Rock has won a certain fame and even adulation because of his efforts, as a Roman Catholic, to persuade the Vatican to approve The ("natural") Pill for birth control. (His own adulation of The Pill is boundless. In the January 1968 *Family Circle,* sold in supermarkets to about seven million housewives, he said that when taken "under the supervision of a competent physician, and directions followed" The Pill "is perfectly safe." No drug "is perfectly safe"; the statement falls in the narrow range between nonsense and non-science.)

Dr. Rock's "natural" theory was too much for physicians who support oral contraception but have not lost their grip on science. Dr. Robert E. Hall of Columbia University, an admitted "birth control enthusiast," termed it "a little short of preposterous." In *The New York Times Book Review* for May 12, 1963, he went on to say, "I would like to dismiss this theory as a harmless euphemism; as a doctor I must aver it is medical fantasy." Does it make any difference if Dr. Rock's theory is "fantasy"? It makes a great deal. There are two reasons, one involving health and the other involving the presumption of The Pill's safety.

1. In a healthy woman the time of peak danger of clotting is following childbirth—the postpartum. If she has one pregnancy after another she can be at maximum risk at most once a year. But on The Pill, the University of Kentucky neurologist Dr. David B. Clark, has pointed out, a woman "is, in effect, pregnant and delivering every month"; and over her child-bearing life she would have "ninety times more chances of showing the complications of pregnancy." In *Child and Family* for Winter 1968 Dr. Herbert Ratner cited a failure to realize that a false pregnancy, a pregnancy without a fetus, is a "disease, not a normal state."

What is ignored in true pregnancy is the compensating factor of a growing and developing fetus, and the adaptability of the mother's body to gestation. . . .

Three examples suffice. In pregnancy, the vascular system of the body adjusts to accommodate a rapidly enlarging uterus. In false or Pill psuedopregnancy, the pelvic vascular system increases the blood supply, but there is no enlarging uterus to utilize the increase. This results in extensive pelvic venous congestion, a condition which has already caused distress to surgeons. Such congestion introduces a whole series of factors predisposing to thrombosis and embolic phenomena.

The second example relates to the hypercoagulable state of pregnancy [i.e., the increased tendency of the blood to clot]. . . . The Pill duplicates the hypercoagulable state. Because it serves no function in false pregnancy . . . The Pill introduces the risk without compensatory advantage.

The third example relates to the well-known protection pregnancy or embryonic tissue confers against certain induced cancers in the lower animal. Projecting this fetal-maternal relationship to human beings, we cannot assume in using The Pill contraceptively, via the mechanism of a false pregnancy, that the protection against cancer is present in the absence of the fetus.

It would seem that if we had any respect for the economies, subtleties and the ordering of health of nature, and any humility in respect to our multiple ignorances of the fetal-maternal relationship to human beings, we would more readily recognize that a state of false pregnancy is pathologic and a monstrosity of nature.

Similarly, Dr. Arnold Klopper, of the Obstetric Research Unit at the University of Aberdeen in Scotland, has said that women on The Pill "are, endocrinologically speaking, in a state of medical castration. . . ." Dr. Frank J. Ayd, Jr., of ment Operations subcommittee, said that the synthetic agents Baltimore, testifying in June 1966 before a Senate Government in The Pill "have multiple effects throughout the body. They resemble the natural ovarian hormones. But, and this is most important, they are NOT the same and therefore cannot be expected to have exactly the same effects. These drugs mimic but do NOT duplicate nature. They cause an un-natural drug-induced state. . . ."

2. An atmosphere in which The Pill is regarded as "natural" serves to inhibit and isolate those who, like Dr. Rivett, the British physician whose poignant plea in the *British Medical Journal* was cited earlier, felt the need for controlled, scientific studies. The atmosphere was one in which the manufacturers could thrive. The oral contraceptives "represent a very considerable financial investment," Dr. Klopper wrote on October 16, 1965, in the *British Medical Journal.* "The commercial interests backing these drugs have at their disposal a formidable machine of medical persuasion. The advertisement campaigns have been designed with great care in order to direct thought along desired lines. It is important to the sale of these drugs that the impression that they create an unphysiological state should not gain ground. *The manufacturers tend to stress the resemblance of their action to the physiological state of pregnancy. They suggest a close relationship between the synthetic gestagens* [progestogens] *and progesterone* [the natural hormone]. . . ."

LEAPING TO CONCLUSIONS

In February 1960 the Food and Drug Administration sent an inquiry to sixty-one professors and associate professors of gynecology and obstetrics: Should it release Enovid, the pioneer Pill, to the market for contraceptive purposes? (The G. D. Searle & Company product had been used since 1957 to treat certain medical conditions, for example, to produce cyclic withdrawal bleeding in women with an absence of menstrual flow.) All sixty-one of the professors replied. Twenty-six—less than half—favored the idea; fourteen "felt that they did not have sufficient data to reach a conclusion," and twenty-one (including at least two concerned with religious considerations) opposed marketing without specifically saying why. Actually, the whole idea of a popularity poll on a complex scientific matter of this kind was not only dubious but also unrelated to the requirement, written by Congress into the Food, Drug, and Cosmetic Act of 1938, that a manufacturer demonstrate the safety of a drug *before marketing* for the uses for which he seeks approval. This had not been done for Enovid, as you will recall from the disclosure that it had been used for a maximum of 38 *consecutive* menstrual cycles in only 132 women. Nonetheless, as noted earlier, the FDA concluded "that the evidence establishes the safety of Enovid tablets for oral use in conception control" and, in 1960, released them to the market.

In 1961 two young women in Los Angeles who had been on Enovid suffered fatal lung clots. Certainly this was news of crucial importance to physicians who were prescribing, or were considering prescribing, Enovid. One such physician was Dr. Henry Olson, clinical professor of obstetrics and gynecology at the University of California School of Medicine in Los Angeles and chairman of the Medical Advisory Committee of the Los Angeles Planned Parenthood Center. "It is interesting to note," he said later, "that I first learned about a fatality, after a patient had taken Enovid—and there had been two in the area of Los Angeles—*from my broker,* who telephoned me one morning and told me the news had come over the wires *from New York* [emphasis supplied]. That was the first time I knew about it." [2]

More such reports continued to be made but attracted scant attention. The situation began to change in the summer of 1962. Although overshadowed by the furor about thalidomide, the baby-deforming sedative, news stories from Britain reported that thrombophlebitis, the painful inflammation of a clotted vein, had occurred in four women on Enovid, and that one of them had died. After a conference with the FDA the Searle firm, on August 7, 1962, sent a "caution" letter to the medical profession in which it said it had reports on twenty-three nonfatal and five fatal cases of clotting among an estimated million users in the United States. The company also said that the diseases can occur without discernible cause, that the available data "neither prove nor disprove a causal relationship," and that any further occurrences should be reported to the FDA and the company. Meanwhile, the American Medical Association reassured the public with a statement that it had made a careful review and found that a causal connection had not been established.

On September 10, 1962, in the hospitable surroundings of the AMA headquarters in Chicago, a conference of thirty scientists was held on the possibility of a link between Enovid —at that time, still the only Pill on the market—and thrombophlebitis. It was not the FDA, the agency that is supposed to protect the public in drug matters, that sponsored the

[2] For another report on The Pill and Wall Street see the cervical case in Chapter III.

meeting but the Searle company; and it was the AMA that conducted the conference. Present as an observer was Dr. Heino Trees, an FDA medical officer. In a memo later, he said that Searle had "reported 132 cases of thromboembolic phenomena among Enovid users, nine of which resulted in death." Apparently, in just a little more than the thirty days since the "caution" letter there had been a surprising surge of reports that raised the number of nonfatal cases from 23 to 123 and the number of deaths from five to nine. Dr. Trees said in a memo:

> A panel discussion was held and general statistical data presented as they were available at that time. The panel, however, *did not make a critical review of the case reports* and expressed the view, with one exception, that the available evidence does not offer any support to the hypothesis that medication with oral contraceptives, especially with Enovid, does contribute to the occurrence of thromboembolic phenomena. To me, as an observer of this meeting, *this resolution was not acceptable, because the decision was based on a statistical answer and yet the statistics one wants to get were unavailable* [emphasis supplied].

To put it another way, the panel of experts lacked the facts on which to base a conclusion but exonerated Enovid; thus they failed to show even the restraint shown by the company which, in the "caution" letter, it will be recalled, said that existing data "neither prove *nor disprove*" a cause-effect association [emphasis supplied].

After only a few hours of discussion of data with immense and potentially grave implications for millions of women and their families, Dr. Michael E. De Bakey called for a vote, saying, ". . . so far there has not been a single shred of evidence that has been presented in any of these figures to suggest that it contributes to a greater incidence of this disease. . . . Will everyone agree with that?" "That it was not unanimous," Dr. Herbert Ratner has said, "is a tribute to Stanford Wessler, M.D., a leading authority on thrombosis, who with courage and perspicacity, was the single dissenting voice."

Within three months after the Searle conference delivered its verdict, the FDA had been told of a doubling of the number of nonfatal cases of thromboembolism, to 242, and of a tripling of the number with fatal result, to 30. Dr. Trees was deeply troubled. In his memo, a copy of which I obtained from other sources, he said that his analysis of the reported cases showed that "the incidence of spontaneous thrombophlebitis, pulmonary embolism and death is higher in the Enovid medicated group than in a similar unmedicated group, convincing me that there is a relationship between this drug and thrombophlebitis. . . . I feel that a critical and urgent reanalysis by a consultant panel is indicated to rule on the safety of this drug by examination of all of the pertinent clinical and statistical data."

On December 18, 1962, the late George P. Larrick, then Commissioner of the FDA, announced that he was appointing an advisory committee to investigate the matter. The group came to be called the Wright Committee, after its chairman, Dr. Irving S. Wright, professor of clinical medicine at the Cornell University Medical College.

IGNORANCE IS BLISS?

The Wright Committee labored for several months, unlike the experts assembled by the Searle company who had needed only several hours to decide that there was not "a single shred of evidence" to show a causal connection between The Pill and clotting. The Committee wanted, first of all, to find out if there was such a connection with *nonfatal* cases. This effort had to be abandoned because, as the committee would say later, "it was impossible to obtain solid comparable statistics." And so the nine consultants concentrated on deaths because "the documentation here would be more complete and valid."

How do you establish the rate at which something occurs? You set up a fraction. For any drug, the numerator is the number of reported cases of the particular adverse reactions with which you are concerned. The denominator is the number of persons who, by taking the drug, were put at risk. If the numerator is too small (because more cases occurred than you know about), or if the denominator is too large (because usage is overstated), or especially if both numerical distortions are present, the incidence understates the reality. In any event, the rate produced by dividing the number of persons at risk into the number of adverse reactions must then be compared with the rate at which these same reactions occur spontaneously—without known cause. Until such a comparison is

made, you don't have a clue whether the drug is responsible
for more reactions than otherwise would occur, that is, for an
excess over normal.

In trying to find out if an excess of fatal vein- and lung-clot-
ting reactions was caused by Enovid in women of child-bearing age, the Wright Committee faced terrific problems. Consider the denominator of women 15 to 45 who in the years at
issue, 1961 and 1962, had used Enovid. No one—not the
manufacturer, not the Food and Drug Administration, not
anybody—knew how many women had been at risk. This
point was driven home by Dr. Arnold Klopper. Writing in
the *British Medical Journal* for October 16, 1965, he said,
"An inquiry to leading companies in this country and in the
United States . . . produced estimates varying from five million to 20 million women all over the world taking these
compounds daily." Obviously, a fraction in which the denominator is subject to a variation of 15 million women is a
pretty shaky matter. A second problem was how to deal with
those women who had used Enovid for part rather than all of
a year. A third problem was welfare women who got Enovid
free and then gave the tablets away or picked up extra income by selling them.

The numerator also posed terrible problems. To determine
it for women who did not use Enovid the committee had to
rely mainly on death certificates. Their quality and reliability
vary widely. A surer way to determine if a clot in the lungs
was the cause of death is to autopsy the victim—but an autopsy is done in only 20 to 30 percent of all deaths.

For women known to have used Enovid, the situation was
still worse. The committee relied on a numerator of 12
deaths—the number among Enovid users reported to the
manufacturer and the FDA. But that figure was, and had to
be, a gross understatement. For one thing, a good many doctors do not, and are not required to, tell a manufacturer or
the FDA when a patient on a drug dies; and a good many
are sharply aware that to make such a disclosure on a death
certificate could put a legal weapon in the hands of survivors
who might care to file a lawsuit. For another thing, even
under the best of circumstances—in a hospital of top rank in
which a system has been set up for reporting of adverse drug
reactions—a very large number of such reactions go unreported. This was illustrated in 1965 by Dr. Leighton Cluff
and three Public Health Service epidemiologists. At the Johns

Hopkins Hospital in Baltimore, they made daily inquiries about drug reactions among doctors and nurses in a 120-bed medical service. In addition, throughout the hospital each time a drug reaction occurred a card was supposed to be filled out. But the researchers found that only one reaction in ten was reported. The explanation was that those supposed to fill out the cards failed to so often that throughout the hospital fewer reactions were recorded than the Cluff team had found in their scrutiny of the medical service alone—a 10 percent sample of the hospital. In view of all of this, it is no wonder that in *Life, Death, and the Doctor* (New York City: Alfred A. Knopf, Inc., 1968), Dr. Louis Lasagna of Johns Hopkins charged that the Wright Committee's reliance on the fatality records in the files of G. D. Searle & Co. was an "appalling mistake." But that mistake was only the first of several. The others he listed included the use of death certificates—"notorious for their inaccuracies"—as another statistical underpinning, and "crystal-ball gazing" that resulted in the subtraction of an even 300,000 from the number of estimated users (mainly to eliminate refill prescriptions) and a "selective discarding"—a generous phrase—of three deaths among Enovid users in the testing in Puerto Rico, where the dead usually are buried within 24 hours.

Knowing such facts about the Wright Committee study, would *you* draw any big conclusions from it? Of course not. In truth, the committee didn't draw any, either. What it did say was that on the basis of the data available to it—*data that were full of holes*—it had judged "an incidence of death among all Enovid users of 12.1 per million cases and an adjusted incidence rate of 8.4 per million in the general population, the difference not being statistically significant." There isn't any doubt that a difference of 3.7 deaths per million users may not be statistically significant, but, as Elinor Langer pointed out on August 16, 1963, in *Science,* "if only 10 percent fewer patients took Enovid than the committee calculated, it is reported, the death rate from the drug would come very close to statistical significance for all ages; and if 50 percent fewer people took it, the rates would be very significantly greater."

Although the Wright Committee warned that "any firm reliance on the risks as calculated is tempered by the assumptions made," and although it said that in the absence of "comprehensive and critical studies" a causal relationship with clotting "should be regarded as neither established nor excluded," the consultants nonetheless spoke a few magic words that tended to undermine the cautious language. These words were: ". . . no significant increase in the risk of thromboembolic death from the use of Enovid in this population group has been demonstrated." As at least some members of the committee must have known, these were the words that would be seized upon by news media, by manufacturers, and by everyone else with a stake in perpetuating the notion that the safety of The Pill had been affirmed by distinguished scientists retained by the government of the United States. Enovid sales boomed. Within a year the number of regular users increased by an estimated 1.7 million.

The hosannas which greeted the Wright Committee report obscured a crucial point: that in frank recognition of the miserable statistical swamp in which it had found itself, the committee had made one, and *only one*, recommendation. This was that "a carefully planned and controlled prospective study be initiated with the objective of obtaining more conclusive data. . . ." The committee was, to put it another way, pleading for a scientific study that would yield the facts from which conclusions could be drawn. In a prospective, or looking-forward study, as has been noted earlier, women would be divided at random into groups on The Pill and groups on conventional contraception or no contraception at all, so that the incidence of disease could be obtained and compared.

GOVERNMENT FOR THE PEOPLE?

Three years *after* the Food and Drug Administration had concluded that Enovid was safe and let it go on the market, a committee of experts appealed for a study to find out if Enovid was, or was not, safe. That such a study was not made *before* Enovid went on sale disgraces the manufacturer, but even more it disgraces the government of the United States because it is on the agencies of the government that citizens who are helpless in matters such as these must depend for protection of their interests. I speak not only of the FDA, which put the urgent recommendation of the Wright Committee on the shelf and which could not avail itself of the excuse that it lacked funds because it never asked Congress for funds. I also speak of the Department of Health, Education, and Welfare, the White House, and the Congress, all of which failed to put the FDA on the spot for putting out of sight and out of mind the advice of the committee whose advice it had sought. But I want to give particular attention to the FDA's sister agency in the Department of Health, Education, and Welfare, the National Institutes of Health. Although the NIH are funded at the rate of about one billion dollars a year, their order of priorities was such as not to provide, until very late in the game, the minimal sums needed to ascertain in a scientific manner whether the constantly growing use of The Pill was endangering millions of American women. In 1962, when the Wright Committee was saying that a prospective study on clotting was a critical and urgent need, the NIH discussed but did not attempt such a study. The estimated cost of the study, which would have provided *real* answers by 1965, was 2.5 million dollars. This was a fraction of the annual profit of G. D. Searle & Company, but neither Searle nor any other manufacturer was willing to sponsor a study of this kind.

The other major type of scientific study is retrospective, or looking backward. In the case of The Pill and clotting, this means essentially that investigators using accepted screening and interviewing techniques compare matched groups of women who have had the disease to see if the rate of occurrence is higher in users than nonusers. The prospective method is more accurate and far more likely to pinpoint a cause-effect association if there is one. However, a careful, well-planned retrospective trial is infinitely to be preferred over no trial at all. The NIH sponsored no study of this type, either. The job ultimately was done—superbly—by the British, who found a seven to tenfold increase in fatal and serious clotting in women on The Pill; and on the basis of the British studies, not on the basis of any work whatsoever in our billion-dollar-a-year NIH, the danger at last was recognized and the labeling changed. This dismal record of nonperformance by the NIH is not wiped clean by the fact that in 1967, seven years after The Pill entered the market, the National Institute of Child Health and Human Development entered into a contract with the Kaiser-Permanente Medical Care Program in and around the Oakland, California, suburb of Walnut Creek for a prospective study. The first intake of volunteers did not begin until early in 1969.

THE BURDEN OF PROOF

Nobody—not the Food and Drug Administration, not the National Institutes of Health, not the American Medical Association, not the Wright Committee, certainly not the conference sponsored by G. D. Searle & Company—interfered significantly with the rising tide of popularity of The Pill and the rising tide of profits to be made from it. The FDA let more formulations and brands enter the market; but having set disastrously low standards for the entry of Enovid it could not—or so, apparently, it was felt—abruptly set substantially higher standards for rival brands. Meanwhile, troubled but isolated physicians kept reporting cases not only of clotting diseases in the legs, pelvis, and lungs, but also in the blood vessels of the brain—strokes. On June 6, 1963, for example, a 23-year-old airline stewardess arrived in London on a flight from the United States during which she had two episodes of feeling unreal and having a sensation of falling. On landing, Dr. K. J. Zilkha reported later in the *British Medical Journal,* she was confused and had difficulty with her speech. Two hours later, in a hospital, "she was disorientated and had difficulty in naming objects. . . . She showed weakness of the right side of the face and weakness of the right hand." She had, of course, suffered a small stroke, or cerebrovascular episode, which kept her in the hospital for a month and from which she subsequently recovered. In discussing the stewardess and also a 26-year-old woman who began to notice "something" wrong with her vision, Dr. Zilkha pointed out that in each case the patient had begun using Enovid only a short time before. He avoided drawing a conclusion because "it is, of course, true that even young people can, rarely, have cerebrovascular lesions from no apparent cause." Dr. Zilkha's report stimulated others. One was made in the *British Medical Journal* about six weeks later, on December 12, 1964, by Dr. A. M. Stewart-Wallace of Howe, Sussex, who told of two additional stroke cases in previously healthy women. While a few cases do not "prove any causal relationship," he said, they "add emphasis to the importance of carefully planned prospective studies. . . ."

American physicians were starting to report clotting episodes, too. One, disclosed in the *New England Journal of Medicine* for May 9, 1963, involved a 21-year-old woman who took Enovid, developed marked fatigue six weeks later, and then suffered a massive pulmonary embolism. She survived. Within fourteen months—a short period in matters of this kind—six cases of lung clotting in women on Enovid were encountered in a single institution, the Henry Ford Hospital in Detroit. In the *Journal* of the American Medical Association for May 11, 1964, a cautious suggestion was made by Drs. Irwin J. Schatz, Roger F. Smith, Gerald M. Breneman, and George C. Bower: that The Pill "may rarely cause thromboembolism in susceptible individuals," and that the possibility of a causal relation "must be considered until disproved."

A few doctors, however, *were* drawing conclusions and putting them on the record. One of these was Dr. Erik Ask-Upmark of the University Hospital in Uppsala, Sweden. He made a casual survey in which he gathered data on 51 clotting cases, 12 of them fatal. Writing in a leading Scandinavian medical publication in 1966, Dr. Ask-Upmark said, "The burden of proof is certainly up to those who maintain that these preparations are harmless, not to those who, like us, consider that a certain danger cannot be excluded. . . . If any female member of my own family applied to me to get oral contraceptives I would most certainly not dare to give [them] to her."

The trouble was that such cases as those of the airline stewardess and those reported by Dr. Ask-Upmark were as much in search of a genuine scientific study as Pirandello's six characters were in search of an author. Without such a study nothing was established. A mass of scattered observations could no more demonstrate The Pill to be unsafe than a man in public office could prove that he does not beat his wife. Pro-Pill propagandists made the most of the situation with statements implying that proof in medical science is like proof in a court of law—that is, that a drug is "harmless until proven harmful" and that this proof must have a finality which all must concede. Gregory Pincus, the pioneer Pill developer, said that it had yet "to be proved that there is a cause-and-effect relationship" between use of the drugs and the ill effects suffered by some patients. This was tricky and misleading not merely because the legal burden of proof since 1938 had been, as Dr. Ask-Upmark put it, "on those who maintain that these preparations are harmless," but also because such statements cultivated the notion that proof in

medical science can be black and white in nature. Actually,
all that can be obtained is data on *relative* risks. Those with a
responsibility for protecting the public health act on just such
"gray" data on risks, because to insist upon certainty—to
wait for proof that, say, a polluted water supply is causing
typhoid fever—is to risk the public health. Further, no data
ever allow expert statisticians and scientists to say, as did Dr.
Robert W. Kistner in *Postgraduate Medicine* for March
1964, that scrutiny by experts of the available data "has completely exonerated" The Pill as a cause of clotting.[3] The most
that can properly be claimed is that data permit a cautious
finding that between a drug and an adverse reaction there is a
high or low *probability* of a causal association. Had there
been a proper study, then, scientists, albeit with a small
chance of being wrong, could have decided whether clotting
in users of The Pill was occurring at an abnormal rate. Not
having such data, they were unable to cope with those who,
like Pincus, kept saying The Pill had not been proved unsafe
—without ever specifying what degree of evidence would
constitute "proof."

Neither did the Pill advocates concede that "proof" of a
causal connection with serious and fatal clotting diseases perhaps never can be obtained, at least not without violating
medical codes of ethics and the standards of a society in
which a high value is placed on human life. The point is illustrated by migraine headaches, which can signal an oncom-
ing stroke. Some women who may have been prone to migraine but never had it get it on The Pill, lose it when they go
off The Pill and get it again if they resume taking The Pill.
Taking The Pill (or any drug) the second time is called
"challenge"; the reappearance of the side effect is called "response." By established scientific standards, "challenge" and
"response" is powerful evidence indeed of a cause-effect connection. But it is not "proof." And what the proponents such
as Pincus did not tell the medical profession or the public
was not simply that we have to settle for less than "proof" in

---

[3] Dr. Kistner, a member of the faculty at Harvard Medical School,
was quoted in the "Fact Sheet" issued by Searle to book reviewers in
1965 as an attack on my *The Therapeutic Nightmare*. The "Fact
Sheet" also quoted Sir Derrick Dunlop, chairman of Britain's Committee on Safety of Drugs, as saying on September 18, 1965, that any belief that clotting was associated with The Pill "is not as yet proved by
scientific evidence."

the case of *relatively* minor effects such as migraine, but that we have to settle for less than "challenge" and "response" for clotting diseases. To try that exercise when the consequence might be death or lifelong disablement would not be tolerated. It was bad enough for advocates such as Pincus to say that they had not seen "proof" that never could be provided, but it was even worse when the same impossible standard repeatedly was invoked by Dr. Joseph F. Sadusk, Jr., the top doctor of the Food and Drug Administration.

THE "25 MONTH CLUB"

The data vacuum was a lovely climate for promotion of The Pill. Making the most of it, G. D. Searle & Company, among other things, prepared *A Prescription for Family Planning,* a 62-page handbook for "counselors, medical and para-medical groups, educators, clergy and other professionals concerned with marital counseling" and specifically "not available to the general public." The title page of the handbook, which has a Library of Congress Catalog Card Number (64-23200) and other stigmata of supposed scholarship, listed the ten members of an Advisory Council, including Dr. John Rock and two officers of Searle. "Here are some queries about Enovid that scientists have answered and documented," the reader is told. *"Is there a causal relationship between Enovid and thrombophlebitis? /* No such relationship has been demonstrated, say the medical authorities. . . . Investigations were conducted by G. D. Searle & Co., the American Medical Association and the Food and Drug Administration. All reported that there appeared to be no connection between the disease and Enovid."

In the same month the handbook was issued, November 1964, Dr. Irwin C. Winter, Searle's vice president for medical affairs and director of clinical investigation, came to Washington to announce, at a meeting of Alpha Chi Sigma, the professional chemists' society, results of a study that "support" those persons and groups "which held Enovid safe for long-term continuous use." It surely sounded impressive. The study was "closely supervised": physicians conducted it in thirty-eight Planned Parenthood Federation clinics "with the knowledge" of the FDA of the techniques to be followed; more than 10,000 women were participating, and the records on the first 5000 had been "analyzed by computers." This

experiment was, Dr. Winter made it clear, Searle's answer to
the appeal of the Wright Committee for "comprehensive and
critical studies" even though the appeal was made about a
year after the experiment was initiated.

That was more public relations baloney; and the fact that
Dr. Alan F. Guttmacher, president of Planned Parenthood-
World Population, would later describe it in a press release
with phrases such as, "this massive clinical research program"
didn't transform baloney into truth. How could this be? All
those doctors. All those clinics. All those women. How?

At the time Dr. Winter made his announcement, a total of
11,711 women had been examined for enrollment in what
was called the "25 Month Club," a name chosen because the
enrollees were in at least their twenty-fifth month on Enovid.
Of the 5000 patients whose records had been run through
computers, only eight, over an average of nearly three years,
developed thrombophlebitis. This was "very nearly equivalent
to the lowest incidence . . . ever reported in a similar population of women," Dr. Winter said.

There were at least two fatal flaws. Dr. Winter admitted
that there was not "an adequate control group," that is, a
group of comparable women against whom the Enovid patients could be measured. Without controls you have a situation rather like that in the ads which say a certain make of
tire stops "25 percent faster." *Faster than what?* Besides, the
Wright Committee had urged "a carefully planned and *controlled* prospective study" [emphasis supplied]. Dr. Winter's
explanation for the lack of controls in "the most comprehensive large scale study in the oral contraceptive field" was that
an adequate group of nonusers was unavailable because The
Pill "was too popular." This was a breathtaking effort to
snatch a public relations victory from the jaws of a scientific
defeat. So was the glamorization of the phrase "25 Month
Club," so as to mask the second—and still more important
—fatal flaw. This was that in order to be enrolled in the study,
a woman had to have been on Enovid for at least two years,
as has been noted. Thus the study automatically eliminated
the crucially important drop-outs, the undisclosed number of
women who stopped using Enovid, for whatever reason, and
were not among the 11,711 who enrolled. "The patients who
drop out of the trials . . . are much more important than the
patients who stay in them," Professor J. R. A. Mitchell of
Oxford University and the British Medical Research Council

warned at the 1962 conference sponsored by the Searle company. The warning was widely ignored. No attention was given to it in the report on the "25 Month Club" even though the vast majority of the 132 cases that precipitated the conference had occurred *within the first six months of Enovid use.* "No wonder," Dr. Herbert Ratner said in *Child and Family* for Spring 1968, that the Searle-Planned Parenthood study "never found the deaths and the strokes and the multiple pathologies that caused women to discontinue The Pill. . . ." Dr. Ratner pointed out that even though promoters of The Pill had "the earliest and largest clinic experiences" with it, "they were not the ones who discovered and reported serious adverse findings. What was not looked for was not found. What was not surveyed was not seen. What perhaps happened was ignored."

JULIA

On July 12, 1964, *This Week,* the Sunday newspaper supplement, carried an article on The Pill by Dr. Edwin J. De-Costa, attending obstetrician and gynecologist at Passavant Memorial Hospital in Chicago. On the same day, Mrs. J. L. Rhodes, of the Washington suburb of Falls Church, Virginia, recalled later in a letter to President Johnson, her daughter was married. Before dealing with the reasons why Mrs. Rhodes should bother to tell the president about the article, I want to note a few things about it. A subheadline called the piece "authoritative." The American Medical Association endorsed it by means of an inset saying, "AMA Authorized." Dr. DeCosta said, ". . . studies do not indicate that the pills cause clots." *What* studies? To be sure, he said, clots do occur in users of The Pill—but they also occur in women who are nonusers and even in men. In addition to this revival of the problem of camouflage, which I mentioned earlier, Dr. DeCosta offered entertainment: "I am reminded of a recent medical meeting where a doctor reported several instances of leg clots occurring chiefly in patients taking The Pills. Another doctor promptly arose. His patient too had been given a prescription for The Pills, and had developed leg clots. But she had forgotten to have the prescription filled."

There is no entertainment in Mrs. Rhodes's letter.

"Dear Mr. President," she wrote on January 25, 1965. "Prayerfully your attention is called to the sudden and tragic

death of Mrs. Julia Elizabeth Rhodes Cross, age 20, em-
ployed as a file clerk at the Securities Department of the
Navy, at 4:09 P.M. January 6, 1965, at her home, and pronounced dead upon arrival at the Fairfax Hospital."

In the two weeks after the death of Julia, whose nickname
was Judy, Mrs. Rhodes assembled a careful, detailed account
of what had happened. She has authorized me to draw on it
for this book in the hope that it will be of help to others, not
merely by indicating a need for caution but also by helping in
the detection of symptoms of a possible clot. The latter point
is important to women on The Pill because, as the story of
Julia Cross makes clear, medical incompetence can have cata-
strophic consequence even when The Pill need not have. Her
doctor saw her numerous times in a matter of a few months.

The doctor in this case prescribed The Pill for Julia two
months to the day after her marriage. He assured her of the
safety of The Pill and prescribed a supply of Ortho-Novum
tablets in the two-milligram dosage sufficient for six months;
and he asked her to return for an examination at the end of
that time. The prescription was filled four days later, on September 16, 1964. Starting three weeks later Julia became ill
—so ill that in October alone she missed eleven days of work.
She had congestion in her lungs and persistent pain in her
chest and stomach, and the pain spread to her right shoulder
and upper arm, back, and neck. On October 19 she visited
the doctor, her family's physician, for the third time in ten
days. After an examination in which he indicated to Julia a
suspicion that her problem was that someone in her family
was "bugging" her, he sent her home. En route her mother
had to stop the car so she could vomit. Spots of blood were
in it.

In November the doctor, who had prescribed a painkiller,
wrote a new prescription for a different analgesic. On December 23 Julia was able to go to work for the last time. The
next morning, her mother's chronology reports, Julia awoke,
"clawing husband, unable to get breath, pain in chest, afraid
she was going to die. Husband tried to rub back and chest
with Vick's salve, Judy unable to lie down. Called Dr.
———— [and] took Judy in to see him at 9:00. Dr. examined
and assured them it was just a pulled muscle." He wrote a
prescription for a medicine to be taken "for aching or pain
when needed."

Two days later, Mrs. Rhodes' narrative continued, "Judy

no better, in pain, vomiting, sleeping in chair." The doctor directed a doubling in the dose of painkiller. "December 29, Tuesday: Still very ill, much pain, sleeping in chair." Julia was taken to the doctor. He examined her and said that "it was only a pulled muscle. Husband insisted on an X-ray. The Crosses could not understand why the pain moved around stomach, chest, back, arm, shoulder and neck. Husband insisted on an X-ray. Dr. gave Rx for pain. . . .

"December 31, Thursday, Dr.————— called Judy at the apartment 4:00 P.M. and told her the X-ray showed pleurisy and a fluid spot but that he did not know what that was. He called in a Rx. . . ." On January 2 Julia was "no better." Mr. Cross "packed up Judy and all medicine" and took her to a different physician, who "took fluid out of right side of lower chest and taped for ease of pain of breathing." On January 5 Mrs. Rhodes phoned her daughter. "Judy in extreme pain . . . almost impossible to understand her," she recalled. That night, the second doctor "pronounced it pneumonia. . . . She was glad to have pneumonia because they could cure that."

"January 6, 1965, Wednesday . . . Judy phoned her mother at 3:10, said it still hurt but that she was better. Called her husband at 3:20, then went to the TV to change channels. As she bent over she caught her side and cried, 'Oh my Lord what have I done to myself, call Paul.' And that was the end."

Dr. William Enos of the Northern Virginia Doctors Hospital performed an autopsy. His report for the Chief Medical Examiner of the State of Virginia said the cause of death was "multiple pulmonary emboli." Dr. Enos added, "For what it is worth, the decedent had been taking Ortho-Novum, 2 mg., since mid-September 1964."

In her letter to President Johnson, Mrs. Rhodes protested that "newspapers and airwaves are constantly full of information trying to influence the President, Congress, and the general public to give the world contraceptives to curb the population explosion." She wondered how many deaths are "attributed to other causes. . . . How many autopsies are performed in . . . India or even in Virginia, U.S.A.?" Mrs. Rhodes enclosed a copy of the article by Dr. DeCosta in *This Week,* noting that it had appeared on the day of her daughter's marriage. She told me she did not know what role, if any, it may have played but said she had found it in Judy's files. "We sorrow not as others who have no hope but while in grief over our own loss pray that God's high purpose will be accomplished and others may be saved," Mrs. Rhodes told Mr. Johnson.

The letter was referred to the FDA. On February 26, 1965, then Deputy Commissioner John L. Harvey, offering "deepest sympathy," wrote to Mrs. Rhodes. Referring to the Wright Committee, he said, "It was the conclusion of our physicians and of the outside experts that the available evidence does not show that the oral contraceptives cause blood clots, and that the drugs are safe for administration under professional supervision. . . . There have been no developments since the expert committee made its study which would alter the earlier conclusion." Harvey was correct. Having ignored the one recommendation made by the committee, for "comprehensive and critical studies," the available evidence remained inadequate to "alter the earlier conclusion."

Mrs. Rhodes is a determined and obviously intelligent woman, and she could not buy Harvey's case. In a letter on May 9 she noted that not until March 23 had an FDA inspector come around to interview her about the extraordinary death of a physically normal 20-year-old woman who had been under "professional supervision." Julia's doctors had access to the "private warnings" in the FDA-approved labeling, but, Mrs. Rhodes wondered, did they *read* them? "Certainly any knowledge of the dangerous side effects would have saved Mrs. Cross as they were *all apparent*," she said. On July 1 the Deputy Commissioner replied. He said that all the materials on Julia's case "have been carefully reviewed" and sounded the old, familiar theme: "There is no adequate evidence yet assembled to show that . . . there is any cause-effect relationship other than that it is coincidental." The second-ranking official in the FDA did not mention that for twenty-seven years the law he was charged with administering put the burden of establishing safety on the manufacturers, not on Mrs. Rhodes and her dead daughter.

The late Justice Robert H. Jackson, in a dissent seventeen years ago in a Supreme Court case (*Dalehite v. U.S.*), eloquently warned us that we are in an era of "synthetic living, when to an ever-increasing extent our population is dependent upon mass producers for its food and drink, its cures and complexions, its apparel and gadgets." He went on to say:

Where experiment or research is necessary to determine the presence or the degree of danger, the product must not be tried out on the public, nor must the public be expected to possess the facilities or the technical knowledge to learn for itself of inherent but latent dangers. The claim that a hazard was not foreseen is not available to one who did not use foresight appropriate to his enterprise.

The only foresight of which I am aware that was appropriate to the great enterprise of The Pill was that shown by those who stood to make money on it.

STROKES AND EYE DAMAGE

Some highlights of 1965:

1. Especially in Britain, physicians—upset, troubled, frustrated by the lack of reliable data—continued to report serious and fatal strokes in healthy young women taking The Pill. In March, Dr. Louis Lasagna of Johns Hopkins disclosed that two colleagues, Drs. David B. Clark (now of the University of Kentucky) and Frank B. Walsh, had collected data on about 20 young women who had suffered strokes, some fatal, after using The Pill. He pointed out that most of these cases had not been mentioned in American medical literature. This disclosure was bracketed in time by Dr. Joseph F. Sadusk, Jr., director of the Bureau of Medicine of the Food and Drug Administration. In 1964—in the July 3 issue of *Life*—his message to the women of America had been, "We are not taking a *dogmatic* attitude that oral contraceptives are *absolutely* safe. . . . But the indications so far are they are safe, when given under the supervision of a doctor . . ." [emphasis supplied]. Now, in 1965, Dr. Sadusk had a fresh supply of pap to dispense. In early April the Committee on Safety of Drugs in London, an official agency, publicly urged physicians in the United Kingdom to report all cases of strokes in women on The Pill. Dr. Sadusk's comment was, "It seems reasonable to conclude at this time that there is no evidence of a cause-and-effect relationship. . . ." There was not "proof," but there *was* "evidence." Dr. Sadusk went on to say that the "information at hand is to the contrary." The information may not have been in some literal sense "at hand" for the future vice president of Parke-Davis, but in meetings at the FDA Dr. Sadusk had discussed the informa-

tion on strokes and The Pill which the *British Medical Journal* had been publishing starting in 1962; and that information *was not "to the contrary."* Neither, of course, were the data gathered by Drs. Walsh and Clark. Within days after Dr. Sadusk made that incredible statement it was knocked in the head by a report from the University of Miami School of Medicine, the difference being that Dr. Sadusk was widely reported while, except for a fine job by the *Miami Herald,* the report from Florida was not. The report—made initially at Jackson Memorial Hospital in Fort Lauderdale and later, in a full-dress version, before the American Heart Association— was prepared by Dr. Sherif S. Shafey, who heads the Cerebral Vascular Research Center, and Dr. Peritz Scheinberg, chairman of the Neurology Department. The report dealt with women who had had strokes and had been taking The Pill for between six months and three years. The researchers found "a strong suggestion of an increase in the number of young females" having such episodes and—in stark contrast to Dr. Sadusk—urged "awareness of the possible existence of a causal relationship."

2. On November 13 in *Lancet,* D.A. Cahal, Medical Assessor for Britain's Committee on Safety of Drugs, reported that among an estimated 400,000 women who had used The Pill through the full year ended August 31, eight had died from clots in the lung. This was *four times* the rate expected, on the basis of mortality statistics for women between the ages of 15 and 45 in England and Wales. Cahal said that "no firm conclusion can be drawn," but it could not be denied that a rate of fatal pulmonary embolism of two per 100,000 among users of The Pill as compared with 0.5 among nonusers, was statistically *highly* significant. This was a severe attack on the validity of the finding by the Wright Committee of a "not . . . statistically significant" difference of 1.21 per 100,000 among Enovid users and of 0.84 among nonusers. The lung-clot comparison in Cahal's report got little attention—none, so far as anyone knows, from the policymakers in the FDA.

3. The agency was busy, meanwhile, throwing up another smokescreen. This one involved the computer mystique— someone says "computer," and you are supposed to bow down and pitch your common sense into the wishing well. In October, the FDA said that a computer was "memorizing" more than 10,000 instances of "adverse experiences" with The Pill. This was said to be part of an FDA "crash pro-

gram" to catalogue every scrap of information available on The Pill—an inadvertent acknowledgment that its surveillance of adverse effects was, contrary to claims made to congressional subcommittees and to survivors of victims such as Julia Cross, in need of strengthening. Actually, the 10,000 reactions were a mixed bag of often sketchy reports in medical journals, of cases from manufacturers' files, of cases reported by private physicians with uneven care and precision, of cases unreliably reported from a small proportion of the nation's hospitals. A truly prophetic warning came at about this time from Dr. John T. Litchfield, Jr., a drug industry scientist, in a speech at dedication ceremonies for the FDA's new building. He said that many people in industry had been "learning a few hard facts of life" about computers. " 'Gigo' is the word—garbage in, garbage out. Computers cannot improve data."

4. In April—the month in which the FDA's top doctor was concluding that the available evidence did not indicate a causal relation between The Pill and cerebrovascular accidents —the *Archives of Ophthalmology* published an appeal to eye doctors to report cases of women on The Pill who had suffered visual troubles. The appeal was made by Dr. Frank Walsh, professor emeritus of ophthalmology at Johns Hopkins. As noted, he already had encountered such troubles, as well as strokes. The results of his appeal did not demonstrate a causal relation; nonetheless the eye doctors, who would see only a fraction of those women with troubles on The Pill, quickly reported injuries involving blood clotting in sixty-one women, including seventeen with strokes, twenty-one with eye problems, and twenty-three with migraine and other symptoms. The results were published in the November issue of the *Archives* with a recommendation by Dr. Walsh for further study and a request that additional reports be submitted to the FDA. In a statement on November 16, the FDA said it had been "privileged to see this paper in manuscript form *several months ago*" [emphasis supplied]. But it did not tell the medical or lay publics about it during that period. The statement recalled that even though a cause-effect association had not been shown, the FDA had, in May, gotten a warning about vision problems into the labeling for Eli Lilly & Company's C-Quens, which then were entering the market. This created another of those crazy situations where a doctor could be led to believe that a particular hazard was peculiar

to one brand, whereas the hazard in fact was no more or no less present in that brand than in others. The FDA explained that it had planned to require the vision warning in the labeling for all versions of The Pill, but had delayed in the expectation that an Advisory Committee on Obstetrics and Gynecology could be convened at an organizational meeting in September. "Since it has not been possible to convene such a committee until November 22-23, 1965, a decision was reached approximately thirty days ago . . . to request manufacturers to incorporate such labeling during the interim. . . ." Once again the camouflage was dragged over all clotting and eye abnormalities in women on The Pill: "It should again be noted that these are naturally occurring conditions which have appeared in women as long back as medical experience goes." It should be noted here that on December 12, 1967, at the annual meeting of the American Academy of Optometry, Dr. S. E. Roever told of forty-eight women on The Pill examined for eye symptoms. Nineteen had outward turning of one or both eyes, and twenty had "accommodative losses" resembling that of much older people. In August 1968 in the *Archives of Ophthalmology*, Dr. B. W. Lambert of Harvard Medical School told of changes in the lenses of rabbits exposed to The Pill and said, "The results of this study raise the question of the long-term effects of oral contraceptives . . . on the human lens."

NOT PROVED UNSAFE: THE DOUBLE NEGATIVE

The beginnings of a fundamental change in attitude at the Food and Drug Administration came at the end of 1965, when Commissioner George P. Larrick retired. To succeed him, John W. Gardner, Secretary of Health, Education, and Welfare, picked Dr. James L. Goddard, a vigorous Public Health Service officer. Four days after Dr. Goddard took the oath of office, Dr. Joseph F. Sadusk, Jr., whose role as the FDA's top doctor now was undercut, had a last fling with the American public. On January 21, 1966, he appeared on the Huntley-Brinkley news program on NBC television along with Dr. Louis Lasagna of Johns Hopkins. There was a genuine confrontation over the issues.

DR. LASAGNA: The American public is remarkably unaware of the potential hazards associated with the taking of birth control pills, even for those hazards about which there is little or no controversy.

Ten percent or more of women cannot take these pills for prolonged periods of time because of the development of nausea or severe depression or excessive weight gain or excruciating headaches.

Hundreds of cases have now been observed by physicians in this country and abroad of women who, while taking the Pills, have developed clots in their extremities, in the heart, in their abdomen, in their lungs and brain—and sometimes with fatal results.

It has been difficult to prove beyond all doubt that The Pills are causally related to these incidents. But the clot [cases] I have mentioned, plus the distribution of clots and the magnitude of the clotting seen at autopsies in case studies here and in other institutions abroad, suggest to me very strongly a cause-and-effect relationship.

Furthermore, no one can possibly tell what can be the effects of taking these medications for ten or twenty years more.

DR. SADUSK: I'm afraid Dr. Lasagna is somewhat overcautious in his remarks about the oral contraceptive drugs.

It is true, scientifically speaking, that there is no drug which is safe.

There has been a cause-and-effect relationship demonstrated with the side effects due to the oral contraceptive drugs which we call "minor" reactions. For instance the nausea which results in some patients, the weight gain that is found and the headaches that may develop in certain patients —these are related.

But when we get to the *serious* side effects which have been alleged to be due to the oral contraceptive drugs, there has been no conclusive evidence—and here I include the strokes, the blood clotting, the eye manifestations and the allegations of cancer.

DR. LASAGNA: Frankly, my advice to the American public is to stick to the older, time-tested mechanical methods of birth control unless there are very important overriding reasons for not using them.

DR. SADUSK: Now in my opinion a woman needs to discuss this matter with her doctor to obtain his specific advice. I would see no impelling reason from the standpoint of safety of the drugs at this time for a woman to take other measures rather than the oral contraceptive.

It is our belief in the Food and Drug Administration that these drugs are relatively safe with the data that we have at hand to warrant their continued use under the direction of a physician.

Dr. Sadusk resigned from the FDA in April 1966, two years after he was chosen for the job by Boisfeuillet Jones, former special assistant for health and medical affairs to the Secretary of Health, Education, and Welfare. Before settling on Dr. Sadusk, Jones had said in an interview with the *Evening Star* in Washington that he was looking for someone "acceptable to the industry, the consumers and the academic world"—a noteworthy batting order.

Although Dr. Sadusk's departure was a major event, a still larger one in regard to The Pill followed in August when the Advisory Committee on Obstetrics and Gynecology issued its *Report on the Oral Contraceptives.* The committee had ten members. They were assigned to task forces on various phases of the problem. Each task force wrote a separate paper which was mirrored in the report signed by all ten members. The task force on clotting, headed by Dr. N. J. Eastman, submitted a paper that was in some ways inadequate and weak. For example, where there should have been a bibliography there was instead, for some unknown reason, a reproduction of the caution letter that G. D. Searle & Company sent to doctors in August 1962. A bibliography is standard in scientific papers, and the other task forces supplied them. Much as had the Wright Committee three years earlier, the task force said, "The data derived from mortality statistics are not adequate to confirm or refute the role of oral contraceptives in thromboembolic disease." But unlike the Wright Committee, neither the task force nor its parent Advisory Committee recommended a prospective controlled study —a point sharply protested in a "special report" by Dr. Roy Hertz, a member of the Advisory Committee. One of the reasons given for recommending retrospective studies instead was that prospective studies are "costly to perform." Even if true—and what is the yardstick for "costly"?—the job of an Advisory Committee is to advise what should be done; cost is the proper concern of the FDA and the Congress. In any event, retrospective studies were undertaken, as the committee recommended; and while not complete at this writing, they are expected to be in substantial agreement with the British retrospective studies which, as noted earlier, showed a seven- to tenfold increase in clotting serious enough to kill or send the victim to the hospital.

The overall conclusion about the oral contraceptives was as follows:

> The Committee finds no adequate scientific data, at this time, proving these compounds unsafe for human use. It has nevertheless taken cognizance of certain very infrequent but serious side effects and of possible theoretic risks suggested by animal experimental data and by some of the metabolic effects in human beings.
>
> In the final analysis, each physician must evaluate the advantages and the risks of this method of contraception in comparison with other available methods or with no contraception at all. He can do this wisely only when there is presented to him dispassionate scientific knowledge of the available data.

A "dispassionate" presentation by the committee would have required it to disclose and even to emphasize that the Food, Drug, and Cosmetic Act of 1938 required the manufacturers to provide evidence of safety, and that a finding that The Pill had not been proved unsafe is inconsistent with the letter and the spirit of the law. A "dispassionate" presentation might have noted the oddity of a situation in which in 1960 the FDA held that the safety of Enovid had been demonstrated, while in 1966 the Advisory Committee finds that all formulations of The Pill, Enovid included, have not been proved unsafe. A "dispassionate" presentation would have made the conclusion square with the introduction, where it was frankly recognized that "the difficulty of obtaining such [crucial] data for the oral contraceptives makes unreliable *any assumptions* regarding a cause-and-effect relationship of drug and adverse reaction" [emphasis supplied]. That means The Pill could not be assumed to have been proved unsafe; but it also means The Pill could not be assumed to have been proved safe—as had been assumed by the FDA in 1960. The conclusion of the report was not "dispassionate"; it was a recognition of what was perceived by the committee as a mix of medical and scientific—and social and political—realities.

At a press briefing before release of the report, the chairman of the committee, Dr. Louis M. Hellman, professor and chairman, obstetrics and gynecology, State University of New York in Brooklyn, characterized the document as a "yellow light" of caution. Dr. Alan F. Guttmacher, the Planned Parenthood leader, was quoted in *The New York Times,* as saying the report gave The Pill "a complete green light." Asked about this on a television program in Washington, Committee member Roy Hertz said that any implication of a "green light" was "totally fallacious." But Commissioner Goddard himself, despite sharp, tenacious questioning by Sander Vanocur, recorded a film interview for NBC's *Today Show* in which he misguidedly conveyed to a vast television audience an articulate, authoritative-sounding impression of the safety of The Pill that was much more optimistic and upbeat than the report justified. And so the show was on the road again. The headline on the story in *Newsweek* was "POPULAR, EFFECTIVE, SAFE." On the story in *Time* the headline was, "THE SAFE AND EFFECTIVE PILLS." The Committee had *not* called The Pill "safe," but those media that did surely helped to explain why it was "popular." The *AMA News,* which the American Medical Association calls "The Newspaper of American Medicine," did its part for its physician-readers with a headline saying, "ORAL CONTRACEPTIVES SAFE, FDA SAYS." Although what surely was meant was that no "proof" of hazard had been found, the first paragraphs of two stories, Jonathan Spivak's in the *Wall Street Journal* and Jane E. Brody's in *The New York Times,* said that "no evidence" had been found.[4] Some newspapers, including the morning *Baltimore Sun,* carried no story at all, but their readers perhaps were better served than those who read an advance "dope" story by columnist Carl T. Rowan.

[4] In April 1966 a World Health Organization committee—one heavily influenced by Dr. Joseph F. Sadusk, Jr., of the FDA—issued a report saying that "there is no substantial evidence of adverse reactions to oral contraceptives." But the report nonetheless emphasized needs for research in about twenty different areas, including the pituitary, adrenal and thyroid glands, the ovaries, uterus and vagina, metabolism, mother's milk and congenital anomalies in the offspring of women who had used The Pill. Somehow, Miss Brody could write, and *The Times* could print, on April 9, a story with this initial paragraph: "All evidence indicates that the birth control pills are safe, except perhaps in some special circumstances, an international committee of scientists has concluded."

"I have learned exclusively that, after studying thousands of medical charts and autopsy reports, even with the help of a giant computer, the Committee concluded it had to give 'The Pill' a temporary verdict of 'safe,' " he said. In fairness, however, it should be allowed that Rowan probably was no further off base a few days before the report came out than Dr. Howard A. Rusk was six weeks *after* it was issued. In his Sunday column in *The Times* on September 25, Dr. Rusk began by saying that the FDA committee "concluded that there was no evidence that oral contraceptives were unsafe." He ended by saying that the question " 'Is it safe?' " had been answered "with a positive 'yes.' " [5] Both statements were erroneous.

SAFER THAN CROSSING THE STREET

Early in January 1967, Dr. James L. Goddard, who had been Commissioner of the Food and Drug Administration for a year, was still publicly optimistic about The Pill. "Do you still think The Pill is safe?" Martin Agronsky asked him on *Face the Nation,* the CBS television and radio program. "Yes," Dr. Goddard said. "I believe it is, provided it is taken under a physician's direction and careful consideration is given to all the factors in the medical history." There was, of course, no way in which the most conscientious and skilled physician could take into account a predisposition to clotting which was not evident in that history. If there had been proper research at the outset, a test for such a predisposition might have been devised. This is not a fantasy, as was made

[5] In September 1968 Jack Gould, television columnist of *The New York Times,* said, "If a journalist owns a piece of the action, he should be the first to disqualify himself from editorializing about or discussing any aspect of that business. But if he persists in doing so . . . then at the very least his employer, be it a broadcasting chain or a publisher, should warn a listener, viewer, or reader, of the association, on each and every occasion where it is pertinent." By that admirable standard, *The Times* would have to disclose every time Dr. Rusk discusses drugs, which has been fairly often, that he is the second-ranking editor of *Medical World News,* which derives almost all of its income from drug advertising, and that in behalf of the American-Korean Foundation he has solicited very large donations from the drug industry. Although *Medical World News* has repeatedly been a vehicle for drug ads found by the FDA to be false and misleading, Dr. Rusk said in May 1968, "Drug manufacturers are obliged to and do fulfill their responsibilities to provide the truth, the whole truth, and nothing but the truth regarding their products."

clear in March 1969 by a report in *Lancet*. Three physicians
—Drs. Hershel Jick of Tufts University in Boston, Barbo
Westerholm of the Sweden's Adverse Drug Reaction Committee, and W. H. Inman of Britain's Committee on Safety of
Drugs—said that preliminary but substantial evidence from a
survey of white women in their countries suggested a relation
between certain blood types and clots in the lower body and
lungs. Such clotting was found to be most common in women
with blood types A (42 percent of the population), B (9 percent), and AB (3 percent), but rare in type O (46 percent).

For Dr. Goddard the *Face the Nation* appearance was an
apparent turning point despite his suggestion that all goes
well if you entrust yourself to a physician. That rosy approach was shaken by some hard-nosed questioning by the
panelists. For example, when he was asked whether the experience of 132 women with Enovid for up to 38 consecutive
menstrual cycles was an adequate scientific foundation for
the release of Enovid to the market, the commissioner said it
had been "my impression" that "large-scale studies" had
preceded marketing. "Whether today, if the same problem
came up *de novo*, I would make the same judgment that was
made then, I can't say." From that time on Dr. Goddard
began taking a forthright stand on The Pill. This became obvious on a single day, April 4, 1967, when two important developments occurred, one in Atlanta, Georgia, and the other
in London.

In Atlanta, Dr. Goddard conspicuously chose a meeting of
the American Association of Planned Parenthood Physicians
to warn that adverse reactions to The Pill were being "grossly
underreported," that the lack of adequate data was a "grave
issue," that every doctor should report even the "subtlest experiences" in users, and that each patient should be told
"carefully . . . about all the possible side effects The Pill may
bring on, minor or major." Most major news media ignored
the speech.

In London the Minister of Health, Kenneth Robinson, disclosed in Parliament that the Medical Research Council had
prepared for later release a preliminary report on The Pill
and clotting. He said the report would show "a slightly increased risk." This was a sensational development because it
heralded the end of the dark, seven-year-long era of ignorance about the true nature of The Pill and the ultimate collapse of the very large superstructure of propaganda built

atop that ignorance. The "main message," as *Lancet* called it, was, "that for the first time since oral contraceptives were introduced an authoritative inquiry has shown that they *do* carry an increased risk of thromboembolism." Neither the extremely cautious new attitude of Commissioner Goddard nor the "main message" from Britain were to be found in "Freedom from Fear," a piece of promotion for The Pill which appeared as a cover story in the April 7, 1967, *Time*. There is, said *Time,* in typical ABC (authoritative, brisk, confident) style, "no evidence that the pills cause clots that might travel to the lungs or develop in the brain." It took *Time* eight months to back down—long enough for readers to have forgotten where they had gotten the impression that The Pill offered "Freedom from Fear"—but it did so on December 29, 1967. In a piece with the straightforward headline "THE PILL AND STROKES," *Time* made a 180-degree turn and said sufficient cases had been reported "to convince physicians that there is a cause-and-effect relationship."

The preliminary report of the Medical Research Council to which the Minister of Health had alluded in Parliament was released on May 5, 1967. The key sentence, devastating to the presumption of safety made by millions of women and their doctors, said, ". . . there can be no reasonable doubt that some types of thromboembolic disorder are associated with the use of oral contraceptives." The story rated twelve lines of type in *The New York Times.* The news wire services sent out stories with lead paragraphs that stand out as examples of how a genuine effort by a reporter to be "objective" can produce a grossly distorting result:

LONDON (AP)—The British Medical Research Council says birth control pills may have caused the deaths of 20 women in Britain last year, but riding in a car would have been twice as risky as taking the pills.

LONDON (UPI)—British medical researchers said today birth control pills are not 100 percent safe. But they said The Pill is far safer than a walk across a busy street.

LONDON (REUTERS)—A report in the British Medical Journal linked the death of 20 women in Britain last year with the birth control pill, but said the risk was small compared to the number of deaths in childbirth or in traffic accidents.

Had you been aware that the choice before you was "riding in a car" or "taking the pills"? Had it occurred to you that "walking across a busy street" is a form of contraception? Thus did straight, factual reporting of what the British Medical Research Council itself said help to implant the wild idea that traffic fatalities on busy streets are a sensible yardstick for measuring risks from The Pill, and tend to downgrade that crucial warning—"there can be no reasonable doubt that some types of thromboembolic disorder are associated with the use of oral contraceptives." I do not mean to suggest that the cars-Pills mishmash originated with the Research Council, but I do suggest that the Council put a valued scientific imprimatur on a concept that added nothing but confusion. Pro-Pill propagandists say that such comparisons are useful because they relate incidence rates to ordinary experience and thus bring them within our comprehension. Then why is it that the advocates *never,* so far as I am aware, point out that in the fifty-nine years in which records on polio have been kept, the annual death rate has exceeded 20 per million only twice, while the death rate from clotting among the population taking The Pill was tentatively figured by the Research Council to be 30 per million—50 percent higher? Can a person who considered the crusade against polio to be important argue that clotting on The Pill is unimportant? There is great concern about crimes of violence— murder, forcible rape, robbery, aggravated assault. The incidence of death of white women of child-bearing age from all of these crimes is about equal to a fatal clotting rate of 30 per million in women on The Pill. In 1964 the number of deaths from abortion reported in the United States was 247. ". . . I do not believe that the true total of deaths due to illegal abortion, recorded and hidden, can be much larger than 500 per year," Dr. Christopher Tietze, who favors easing of abortion laws, told the International Conference on Abortion in September 1968. In *Child and Family* for Spring 1968, Dr. Herbert Ratner said, "Most of the supporters of The Pill —the same physicians who are minimizing deaths from The Pill—are in the forefront decrying deaths from illegal abortion as a rationale for relaxation of the abortion laws. They do this with humanistic fervor. All can lament these deaths,

for each human life is precious. But where is their concern
for women dying from The Pill?" [in numbers approximating
those from criminal abortion]. "They dismiss the number of
deaths from The Pill as inconsequential," he continued—but
do not, of course, so dismiss deaths from abortion.

To its credit, the FDA under Dr. Goddard and his succes-
sor as of July 1, 1968, Dr. Herbert L. Ley, Jr., have rejected
the comparison of taking The Pill and crossing streets as a
scientific irrelevancy. And so it is all the more startling and
disturbing that Dr. Louis M. Hellman, chairman of the
FDA's Advisory Committee on Obstetrics and Gynecology,
kept dragging this medical red herring across the television
screens and through the pages of popular magazines. On May
2, 1968, for example, Dr. Hellman appeared on the *Today
Show* on NBC television. "I don't think personally that the
way to talk about this risk of [clotting] is in comparison with
the things we do every day that we don't have to do," he
said. "For example, you don't have to ride in an automobile,"
he said, ". . . and yet the risk of riding in an automobile is
perhaps ten [times higher than the risk of clotting], maybe
even more than that." The good sense award went that day
not to Dr. Hellman but to interviewer Barbara Walters. "But
I could say, Doctor, that in the course of my daily life, I
pretty much have to ride in an automobile," she said. "I can't
walk everywhere, the way cities are today." Can you?

"But I don't have to take The Pill," Miss Walters added.
Do you? Maybe Dr. Hellman's patients, to an unusual extent,
walk, take subways, or swing on ropes tied to the trees that
grow in Brooklyn—I don't know. But, in any case, he was
back making the same argument almost a year later, in the
April 1969 *Redbook:*

> Let's look at some other approaches to the question of risk.
> What are the risks that human beings take every day that
> they don't need to take? One is riding in an automobile—
> you don't need to ride in an automobile. . . . From all the
> available data, we know that the risk in riding in an auto-
> mobile is ten times as great as the risk in taking an oral
> contraceptive. . . . In other words, although the risk in
> using The Pill exists, it is a somewhat minor one.

But for a lot of women the risk is a needless one and by no

means the only one involved. Why does Dr. Hellman seem to
think it important to minimize it?

What about the comparisons so frequently made between
The Pill and the hazards of childbirth? Again there is the
confusion—cautioned against early in this book—that is gen-
erated by talk about women as a monolith rather than as individuals. For a healthy woman to whom high quality medical care is available pregnancy is a much smaller risk than it
is for, say, a woman in the southeastern United States whose
whole family has an annual income of less than $1000,
whose intestinal tract is chronically filled with parasitic
worms, and for whom medical attention of any kind is almost nonexistent. An unmarried girl may regard pregnancy
and abortion as intolerable—but the girl who will reliably use
vaginal foam or a diaphragm with vaginal cream or jelly
must be distinguished from the girl for whom The Pill is the
only reliable form of contraception. Surely these observations
may strike you as being as protuberantly obvious as the abdominal profile of a woman nine months after conception.
Yet there persist comparisons of the hazards of pregnancy
with The Pill that are so generalized as to be almost meaning-
less for individual women—if I may say so once more, for
you, for your daughter, your sister, your friend. Such comparisons can be further biased by a failure to recognize that
pre-existing poor health "contributes to most of the deaths in
pregnancy," as Dr. Ratner has said. "Contrasting the death
rate of healthy women on The Pill to healthy pregnant
women results in an entirely different comparison." Similarly,
Dr. Louis Lasagna found in the report made in 1966 by a
committee of the World Health Organization "an interesting
and subtle point: Many doctors will not prescribe oral contraceptives in women with a history of thromboembolic disease. Thus in a sense The Pill is being given to healthier
women than the average population, possibly biasing present
risk estimates in favor of The Pill."

Even if these important considerations are put aside, fallacies can be exposed in comparisons of the kind made by various supporters of The Pill, including Joshua Lederberg, win-
ner of a Nobel Prize in 1958, and Dr. Hellman. This is an
argument Lederberg made on September 18, 1966, in the
Washington Post: ". . . even today pregnancy carries a risk
of 300 maternal deaths per million gestations. This number is

at least 20 times higher than for any specific side effects that might conceivably be attributed to The Pill by interpretation of the existing statistics."

Lederberg was saying that the risk of fatal clotting among one million women on The Pill could not possibly exceed one-twentieth of 300, or 15; but, a matter of months later, the British Medical Research Council was estimating twice that number (30 deaths per year in excess of normal on the basis of three deaths per year among 100,000 women using The Pill).

A different approach was used by Dr. Hellman in the article in *Redbook* and again in *The New York Times Magazine* last July 20. This is what he said in *Redbook:*

> If we take a model population of 100,000 fertile women, all married to fertile men and using no contraception, they will have 50,000 babies at the end of a year. And there will be, according to the current maternal death rate in the United States, 15 deaths. (These deaths are caused by complications during pregnancy or childbirth.) If these women use diaphragms, they will have 10,000 babies (the diaphragm has a 10 percent failure rate), and they will have, in proportion, three deaths. Finally, if you prescribe oral contraceptives to these 100,000 women, very few of them will have babies, but three of them will die from using the oral contraceptives. So it can be said that The Pill is as safe (or as dangerous) as the diaphragm.

Yes, that can be said, and Dr. Hellman has said it, but it isn't so. As Dr. Hellman must know, the 10 percent failure rate he ascribes to the diaphragm has nothing to do with reality for those women—probably including a good many readers of *Redbook* and *The Times Magazine*—who use the diaphragm consistently and properly and risk, say, the one percent failure rate listed by Dr. Waldo Fielding. Among a group of such women deaths would number 0.3, or, to put it another way, three in ten years, not three in one year. That's quite a difference, but there's more to be said. Take the death rate in the age group 35 to 44. Months before Dr. Hellman's article appeared, the FDA labeling listed the fatality rate not as three per 100,000, but as 3.9 (two and one half times the 1.5 for the 20-to-34 age group). Although the ebullient Dr.

Hellman slighted it, that same official labeling shows that among the 100,000 women on The Pill, 47 per year will have clots in the lower body, lungs, or brain serious enough to send them to the hospital and to leave some of them permanently disabled.[6] In addition, Dr. Hellman's "model" also brushed off the risks from multiple other diseases associated with The Pill.

The commonest and worst form of statistical manipulation has been premised on plausible but deceptive reasoning that goes like this: Take 1,000,000 women. If all become pregnant 300 will die (for Britain the figure used by the Research Council was 120, which incidentally may tell us something about the overall quality of health care in the two countries); but if all used The Pill (this assumes complete efficacy) only 30 would die. Therefore The Pill has saved 270 (90 in Britain) women from maternal mortality. By now it should be crystal clear, however, that such a comparison can have validity only for those women who can be depended upon to consistently and properly use no form of conception control but the combination form of The Pill. For women who reliably will use, say, vaginal foam or a diaphragm with spermicidal jelly or cream, such a comparison is as trickily irrelevant and misleading as a comparison with traffic accidents. This is easily demonstrated. Let us assume for such women a failure rate of 1.5 percent for the diaphragm or foam. Obviously it is not the 1,000,000 women in the statistical sample who are exposed to the hazards of maternity, because only 1.5 percent of them, or 15,000, become pregnant. The rate at which maternal mortality occurs, 300 per million, must be applied, consequently, to the 15,000. The computation shows that four or five (4.5) women will die—at least 25 fewer than the 30 fated to die from clotting among the 1,000,000 taking the combination Pill. The sequential Pill would fare even worse in an analysis of this kind, because in addition to the 30 deaths from clotting there would be a few more fatalities re-

6 All of these clotting rates were adapted by the FDA from the British studies reported on April 27, 1968, in the *British Medical Journal,* for the years 1964–66. Last June 14 this journal published a new report in which Drs. M. P. Vessey and Richard Doll presented data on hospitalization rates in 1967. Their conclusion was that the "best quantitative estimate" was still higher—50 per 100,000 for users compared with six per 100,000 for nonusers.

sulting from maternal mortality in the tens of thousands of women in whom it failed to prevent conception. Once again, the poor showing of both types of The Pill in this analysis is an understatement because it does not take into account non-fatal clotting and other hazards.

But the suggestion was made most anywhere you looked that The Pill was the only way to avoid pregnancy. In 1967, for example, Ernest Havemann said in *Birth-Control,* a Time-Life book, that the risks of clotting from The Pill "are far less than those of an ordinary pregnancy." In Parliament, Health Minister Kenneth Robinson emphasized the larger "total risks associated with pregnancy." In the *Sunday Times* of London, Moira Keenan—using British maternal mortality figures, of course—said that although 30 clotting deaths per year may occur among 1,000,000 users of The Pill, "four times this number could die from thrombosis if they became pregnant." In 1968 Dr. Louis M. Hellman, the FDA's top consultant, said on May 2 on the *Today Show,* "The British say the risk is less than having a baby. *Perhaps* this isn't the proper way to evaluate the risk" [emphasis supplied]. There is no "perhaps" about it. It was at this point that Dr. Hellman went on to suggest that the "proper way to evaluate the risk" was to compare it with "the risk of riding in an automobile." At about the same time, *The New York Times* reported that the 1968 British studies "noted that the risk attributed to the Pills was substantially less than the risk of death from pregnancy." And *Newsweek* called attention to the "well-established risk of blood-clot complications in pregnancy." In October 1967 *Parents' Magazine* carried an article purporting to show that The Pill could not cause clotting at all. This point could be persuasive provided data on clotting episodes were used without acknowledgment that the reported episodes are but a fraction of the total which actually occur. And so the fact of underreporting was not disclosed to the readers of *Parents',* even though underreporting had been admitted in March 1965 in *Metabolism* by an executive of G. D. Searle & Company, Dr. Irwin C. Winter. The author of the *Parents'* article, Dr. George Langmyhr, medical director of Planned Parenthood-World Population, was formerly associated with Ortho Pharmaceutical Corporation. The data on which he relied were taken from *Oral Contraceptives,* a book by Dr. Victor A. Drill. Dr. Drill is director of biological research for Searle.

MORE ON STROKES

The preliminary report from Britain in May 1967 found "no reasonable doubt" about an association between The Pill and clotting in the lower body and the lungs, but was tentatively less certain about a relation with clotting in the bloodways of the brain. And, it will be recalled, strokes did not figure in the Wright Committee report of 1963; and in April 1965 Dr. Joseph F. Sadusk, Jr., was assuring the public that he had at hand "no evidence" of a causal association with strokes—indeed, that his information was "to the contrary." However, the year 1967 brought several most disturbing new reports, including these:

MARCH 25—Drs. Edwin R. Bickerstaff and J. MacDonald Holmes, writing in the *British Medical Journal,* said that their clinical experience over a 13-year period suggested "an apparent association" between The Pill and strokes. In the 10 years ending in 1963, in the Birmingham region, these neurologists had seen 25 previously healthy women of child-bearing age who had suffered strokes of undetermined origin. These cases averaged two or three a year. This indicated that in the years 1964 through 1966 a total of six or eight new cases would be referred. And there were in fact referred to Drs. Bickerstaff and Holmes seven women who had unexplained strokes—and who had not been using The Pill. But in the same years, years of greatly increased use of The Pill, they also treated 18 other previously healthy young women —13 were under 35—for unexplained strokes. All of the 18 "had been taking one or other of the oral contraceptives," half of them for less than nine months, some for as little as three months and some for as much as two years.

One of the victims suffered paralysis in the left arm and left side of the face four months after going on The Pill, made a partial recovery, disregarded advice to stop using The Pill, and, six months later, abruptly suffered impairment of the power to use words to express herself and paralysis of the right arm. Within a week she made a partial recovery but was beset by involuntary laughing and crying. Finally, she began to make steady recovery. A woman of 30 had taken The Pill for a year when she began to suffer visual problems. "On two occasions she suddenly fell to the ground, probably without impairment of consciousness, but once with vertigo," the article said. She refused to go off The Pill. The attacks continued. After three months "she finally agreed to stop the oral contraceptives but two days later suddenly died.' (The cover story on The Pill in the subsequent April 7 issue of *Time,* it will be remembered, said that there is "no evidence that the pills cause clots that might travel to the lungs or develop in the brain.")

APRIL—In a paper given at the annual meeting of the American Academy of Neurology in San Francisco, three neurologists from Western Reserve University School of Medicine in Cleveland said that migraine headaches, especially if accompanied by visual difficulties, can be the signal of impending serious complications, including strokes, in users of The Pill. The physicians—Drs. John H. Gardner, Stanley van den Noort, and Simon Horenstein—said that in such circumstances a woman should stop use of The Pill. They concluded that migraine could be the herald of stroke on the basis of their study of nine young women at the University Medical Center who had been on The Pill, who had suffered strokes, and who in each case had had a migraine before the stroke. Of the approximately 200 neurologists who heard the paper, an estimated two-thirds raised their hand when asked if they had seen Pill users who had suffered strokes preceded by migraine. An abstract of the paper referred to the nine cases as "drug-induced catastrophes." Also in April, Dr. Harold Stevens, head of the Department of Neurology at George Washington University School of Medicine in Washington, told me in an interview that ". . . it appears that some undetermined increase in cerebrovascular accidents has occurred as a result of the contraceptive pill."

NOVEMBER—In the *Archives of Internal Medicine,* Dr. Monroe Cole, of the Department of Neurology at Bowman Gray School of Medicine in Winston-Salem, North Carolina, reported on six cases of brain damage in young women, two of them 24-year-old mothers of young children, who had been on The Pill. "A stroke in a young woman is an uncommon clinical event," Dr. Cole said, and ". . . we have been impressed with the fact that we are seeing a greater number of young women with strokes in the past year than we had been seeing previously. . . . The evidence is sufficient to cause the medical profession to weigh carefully the indications and possible alternatives before prescribing these drugs. . . . If the public were more aware of the possible dangers, alternative methods of contraception might become more acceptable."

A year later a surprising point about the clinical profile of strokes in young women on The Pill was made by Dr. F. A. Elliott, of the Pennsylvania Hospital in Philadelphia, in the *Journal* of the American Medical Association. This profile often differs "significantly from the cerebral vascular accidents of young people in the pre-'Pill' era," he said in a report on December 16, 1968, on three illustrative cases he had treated. "In the first place, the localization and clinical characteristics of the stroke itself are often bizarre. Secondly, the duration of incapacity is unusually brief. Thirdly, no further incidents occur if the patient shuns the Pill." He said he was left with "a strong impression that we are witnessing the appearance of a new 'disease' which is separate and different from the strokes which sometimes develop in young people. . . ."

THE BRITISH STUDIES

On January 18, 1968, at a press briefing in Washington, Dr. Louis M. Hellman, chairman of the Advisory Committee on Obstetrics and Gynecology of the Food and Drug Administration, officially recognized for the first time the existence of a cause-effect relation between The Pill and clotting in the legs, pelvis and lungs. He had, he said, been given the final results of final British studies in confidence and hence could not divulge them; but the results would soon be published in the *British Medical Journal*. How striking a commentary it is not merely on our national priorities, but on our priorities within medicine, and on our constant emphasis on *new* drugs, *new* techniques, that the definitive tests on the safety of The Pill were undertaken in Britain. The Pill "was first discovered, researched, clinically tested, marketed and widely used in the U.S.," Dr. Herbert Ratner said in *Child and Family* for Spring 1968, ". . . and although the number of women in the U.S. far exceeded use in other countries, and although there were four U.S.-dominated committees appointed to look into safety, it was not the U.S. with its much vaunted scientific resources and superior health accomplishments that resolved this vital question. It was resolved by England, a medically socialized country whose resources, supposedly, do not compare to ours." At the press briefing, which had been called for another purpose, Dr. Hellman said that the risk demonstrated by the British studies was "very, very small"— a view he repeated on May 2, 1968, on the *Today Show,* following publication of the British studies; in addition, he told the NBC television audience that The Pill "has proved remarkably safe. . . ." The British studies were conducted by Drs. W. H. W. Inman and M. P. Vessey for the Committee on Safety of Drugs, and by Drs. Vessey and Richard Doll for the Medical Research Council. Their reports appeared in the *British Medical Journal* for April 27, 1968. Both reports were the products of retrospective studies—the Inman-Vessey paper of 1,024 cases of clotting which occurred after The Pill or other hormonal preparations had been ingested, the Vessey-Doll paper of cases and controls treated in 1964–66 in large general hospitals.

In the Inman-Vessey mortality study, in which the controls were comparable patients in the practices of the reporting physicians, 88 reports referred to a fatal outcome, but a smaller number, 53, were found to have involved known users of The Pill. Of the 53, 36 involved "excess" deaths in which The Pill alone was the suspected cause. Highlights of the study are as follows:

● Only eight of the 53 Pill deaths had been reported to the Committee on Safety of Drugs, making "untenable" the assumption—which underlies the claim that no causal relation exists—that reporting of such deaths is almost complete.

● The data establish with a "great disparity" of "excess" deaths a "statistically highly significant" cause-effect relation with fatal clotting in the lungs.

● The evidence for a causal relation with fatal strokes, which are believed to involve the cerebral arteries rather than the veins, "is also strong . . . and it seems reasonable to conclude that a small but definite risk exists."

● ". . . irrespective of age, the risk of death from pulmonary embolism or cerebral thrombosis was increased seven to eight times in users of oral contraceptives."

● Among women age 20 to 34 the mortality attributable to The Pill was 15 per million, compared with two per million among nonusers, for an "excess" of 13 deaths per million users per year. (I am using a base of a million rather than 100,000 simply to avoid decimal points here.)

● Among women 35 to 44 the mortality rate attributable to The Pill was 39 per million, compared with 5 per million among nonusers, for an "excess" of 34 deaths per million users per year.

● Among some subgroups in the study there was a "a significant association between oral contraception and death from coronary thrombosis" (heart attacks). Although the data did not "quite" attain statistical significance, Drs. Inman and Vessey were troubled by them to the extent that they reported what the mortality figures would be with the statistics on heart attacks included: 22 per million per year in women age 20 to 34, and 45 per million per year in women 35 to 44. (The uncertainty about oral contraceptives and heart attacks shown by these distinguished researchers has induced considerable wariness in me. In the *British Medical Journal* for June 14, 1969, Drs. Vessey and Richard Doll, taking into account supplemental evidence which became available after the 1968 report was published, said that it fails "to provide any indication that they also cause coronary thrombosis.")

● If the risk attributable to the use of oral contraceptives is expressed in terms of the total risk of death [in the child-bearing age span of 20 to 44] this risk amounts to about two percent of the total mortality."

● "It is probable . . . that all these estimates of risk are too low because information from independent sources indicates that our control data substantially overestimated the use of oral contraceptives by the general population in 1966." That is to say, an overestimate of use of The Pill in the control, or yardstick, population artificially reduces the number of "excess" deaths among users in the test or Pill-using population. Figuring the overestimate to be almost 40 percent higher than it should have been, Drs. Inman and Vessey said that it "seems very likely that we have *underestimated the mortality attributable to contraceptives by a similar amount*" [emphasis supplied].

• "On balance, it seems reasonable to conclude that the risk from pulmonary embolism during one year's treatment with oral contraceptives is of the same order as the comparable risk of bearing one child. In assessing the risks, however, it is important to remember that women in the United Kingdom give birth, on average, to only two or three children in their lifetime, that other methods of contraception are reasonably effective, and that birth control may be practiced during most of a woman's child-bearing years."

The Vessey-Doll study dealt with married women aged 20 to 44 who suffered clotting severe enough to require admission to a hospital in 1964–66. Here are the principal findings, supplemented by material in parentheses from a report in the *British Medical Journal* for June 14, 1969, in which Drs. Vessey and Doll took into account data, hitherto unavailable, for the year 1967:

• The annual risk of hospitalization for treatment of all three forms of clotting involved—deep-vein, lung, and stroke —is 470 per million among users of The Pill compared with 50 per million among nonusers. ("The best quantitative estimate of the annual risk of hospital admission for any of the three conditions" is about 500 per million for married women who are using oral contraceptives and about 60 per million for married women who are not).

• The annual risk of hospital admission for deep-vein clotting and pulmonary embolism was the risk clearly established and was "about nine times greater in women who use oral contraceptives than in those who do not." ("The best estimate of the risk of hospital admission for deep-vein thrombosis or pulmonary embolism, in the absence of other predisposing cause, appears to be about six to seven times higher among married women who are using oral contraceptives than among those who are not, with a 95-percent probability of being between 3.4 and 11.6 times higher. Other evidence, derived from national data for contraceptive use by age and parity [in numbers of children borne], *suggests that the true risk is likely to be nearer the upper than the lower of these limits* [emphasis supplied]. This conclusion accords with the estimate derived by Inman and Vessey . . . from mortality data [8.3 times greater] and is compatible with the trends in national mortality statistics [(Vessey and Weatherall . . . Markush and Seigel]. . . .)" [7]

● "From a study of women suffering from cerebral thrombosis, 'taken in conjunction with other similar findings, it is justifiable to conclude that oral contraceptives may also be a cause of cerebrovascular insufficiency' [strokes]." ("The estimate of the risk of [hospital] admission for cerebral thrombosis is less certain, because it is based on smaller numbers; but the best estimate of the relative risk, derived from our data and from the mortality data of Inman and Vessey (1968), *appears to be about the same as that for venous thromboembolism* [emphasis supplied]. Moreover, this is compatible with the hospital experience of Bergeron and Wood. . . .)" [8]

On May 2, 1968, Dr. Louis M. Hellman, the FDA's chief outside consultant on The Pill, was interviewed by Barbara

---

[7] These researchers, to put it bluntly, found where the bodies were buried. In the *British Medical Journal* for July 13, 1968, Drs. Vessey and J. A. C. Weatherall said that the mortality statistics for 1963–67 for England and Wales showed an increase in deaths from clotting diseases in young women on The Pill "of a magnitude compatible with the existence of a causal relation between the use of oral contraceptives and death from venous thromboembolism." In November 1968 Drs. Robert .E. Markush of the National Institute of Neurological Diseases and Blindness and Daniel G. Seigel of the National Institute of Child Health and Human Development announced a parallel finding. In a paper given at a meeting of the American Public Health Association, they said that a comparison of published mortality statistics for the United States in the pre-Pill period and in the usage period of 1962–66 indicated "an association of oral contraceptives with an increase in mortality from diseases of the veins, of which pulmonary embolism is the largest component." Their criterion was "sizable" relative increases in mortality. The Markush-Seigel paper being consistent with all of the British studies, the Food and Drug Administration was left without scientific justification for including in the labeling for The Pill the suggestion that the British data "cannot be directly applied to women in other countries. . . ."

[8] On November 29, 1967, in a paper at the annual meeting in Chicago of the Radiological Society of North America, Drs. R. Thomas Bergeron and E. H. Wood of Columbia Presbyterian Medical Center reported on nine young women who had strokes. Eight had been on The Pill—and half of them had had such likely warning symptoms as severe migraine-type headaches, visual problems, weakness in one side of the body and mild speech difficulties. "We believe that the development of these symptoms should be interpreted as an indication for the immediate and total cessation of the use of these medications," the radiologists said.

Walters on the *Today Show*. He said: "Well, Barbara, I think the British data is [*sic*] *conclusive*. I think that it *proves*—and this is a new item—conclusively, what we've suspected for some time, that there is a cause-and-effect relation between the taking of oral contraceptives and clots."

DR. KISTNER, DR. DRILL, AND SEARLE

Two additional points in the 1969 report of Drs. Vessey and Doll merit emphasis. One was a lack of evidence "that the risk is concentrated during the early months of use or that it increases with increasing duration of use." The second point has to do with an article—prominently displayed in the *Journal* of the American Medical Association for September 30, 1968—that provided evidence that The Pill is *not* a cause of "thrombophlebitis." The article relied on incidence rates in medical literature that indicated close similarities in large groups of users of The Pill and in large groups of nonusers. The article also noted that the recorded incidence of "thrombophlebitis" during pregnancy was unusually low. Drs. Vessey and Doll commented:

> The value of these comparisons is, however, limited, because the series [of studies] were compiled by different workers and the definitions of thrombophlebitis and the completeness of reporting are likely to have varied from one series to another. *Such evidence does not weigh heavily against that obtained by personal investigation of groups of patients under controlled conditions* [emphasis supplied].

The principal author of the article in the AMA *Journal* was Dr. Victor A. Drill, director of biological research for G. D. Searle & Company. The article is relied upon heavily by the pro-Pill Dr. Robert A. Kistner, who quotes it at length in his current book *The Pill: Facts and Fallacies about Today's Oral Contraceptives* and lists it first among his acknowledgments. Dr. Kistner says nothing about Dr. Drill's connection with the maker of Enovid.

Cancer and The Pill III

Our benchmark for talking about a possible association between cancer and The Pill is the report of August 1966 made by the Advisory Committee on Obstetrics and Gynecology of the Food and Drug Administration. This report, it will be recalled, said that the difficulty of obtaining essential data on The Pill "makes unreliable any assumptions regarding a cause and effect relationship of drug and adverse reaction." In other words, the facts on which a scientific judgment of safety could be made are lacking. As to cancer, this was true in 1966 and it is true in 1969. That being so, the fundamental question for patient and physician might well be: Is the need for *oral* contraception so great as to require daily ingestion of potent drugs which may—or may not—have a potential for advancing or causing cancer? Does the physician who prescribes The Pill because a patient wants its convenience observe the medical maxim to first of all do no harm (*primum non nocere*)?

One of the reasons for uncertainty about The Pill and cancer is, as the report emphasized, that "all known human carcinogens [substances that cause cancer] require a latent period of approximately one decade." The Pill not having been approved for contraceptive purposes until 1960, truly widespread use having built up after that, and adequate studies—which require many tens of thousands of women—not having been done, we remain largely ignorant of where this uncontrolled experiment is taking us.

The general assumption was of course that "they"—meaning the government—would not have let The Pill enter the market unless "they" were sure it was safe. Dr. Roy Hertz of the National Institute of Child Health and Human Development inquired of the Food and Drug Administration precisely what evidence it had when it approved Enovid for use in young women for a recommended maximum of four years. On February 4, 1964, Dr. Arthur Ruskin, then acting

88

director of the FDA's Division of New Drugs, told Dr. Hertz in a letter that approval was based on a *four-year experience with 400 women* whose cases were supported by essential laboratory studies. "Since duration of exposure is so critical a factor, only those women exposed for the actually approved period of four years provide any experience pertinent to this evaluation," Dr. Hertz said in an appendix to the Advisory Committee report. "Certainly, it is to be reasonably expected that a new public health practice would be predicated on a more soundly developed epidemiological basis." Dr. Hertz also pointed out that a search of the published medical literature had unearthed data on cancer incidence on a grand total of 85 women who were under 40 and who had taken The Pill continually for four years or longer. Was 85 a sufficient number? I asked Dr. James L. Goddard in January 1967 on *Face the Nation*. "No," he said frankly to a nationwide CBS television and radio audience. "I don't believe it is." On February 17, 1965, Dr. James A. Shannon, then director of the National Institutes of Health, was testifying before a House Appropriations subcommittee headed by the late John E. Fogarty (D–R.I.). The Congressman took up the possibility of a link between oral contraceptives and cancer. There was this exchange:

MR. FOGARTY: So people are really taking a chance.

DR. SHANNON: I believe so. There are a great many studies on experimental animals that indicate that they probably can be taken without hazard, but there has not been adequate human exploration to be certain.

This kind of scientific caution had its heady contrasts, as in the case of clotting. No mention of cancer, one way or the other, was made in most of the pamphlets prepared by makers of The Pill for doctors' waiting rooms. In its February 1966 issue *Good Housekeeping* presented a summary of reasons for concern about The Pill along with a piece entitled "Yes, I'll Still Prescribe The Pills" by Dr. Alan F. Guttmacher, president of Planned Parenthood-World Population. "Although it is too early to draw definite conclusions, there is some evidence to suggest that the combination of progestins and estrogens in the pills may even reduce the incidence of some tumors and retard the growth of others," he said. In April 1967 *Time*, in its "Freedom from Fear" cover story, said,

"Despite dark fears, there is not a shred of evidence that the pills cause cancer. In fact, they may even give some protection against it." This article, which should have established once and for all that *Time* can be just as trustworthy in matters involving the drug industry and favored causes such as population control as in matters involving politics and foreign policy, ignored the report of the Advisory Committee. When the moment of truth came, *Time* took no responsibility on itself but shifted it to others. "The claim was once made that while estrogens may cause cancer, as they do in many laboratory animals, The Pill seemed actually to afford some protection against breast cancer," *Time* said in its May 2, 1969, issue. "More cautious now, *the experts* claim no protective effect . . ." [emphasis supplied].

The case of Dr. Louis M. Hellman, chairman of the Advisory Committee, is a special one. On one hand, he can be moved to strike a cautious note. "There has always been the underlying fear that because the oral contraceptives contain estrogen and estrogen has caused cancer in most experimental animals when used for long periods of time, The Pill might cause cancer in human beings," he said in the April 1969 *Redbook*. "We don't know yet; the risk is still there." On the other hand, there was his statement eleven months earlier on the *Today Show*. After saying substantially what he would say later in *Redbook*, Dr. Hellman was asked by Barbara Walters if he would prescribe The Pill to his own daughter. "Absolutely," he said.

This is what the Advisory Committee said about animal studies in re cancer:

Sex steroids, particularly estrogens, have been shown to produce malignant lesions and to affect adversely the existing tumors in the mouse, rat, rabbit, hamster and dog. These neoplasms [new growths] have occurred in various organs, such as the cervix, endometrium, ovary, breast, testicle, pituitary, kidney, and bone marrow. . . . Animal studies in which certain susceptible strains and species are used and in which the dosage is excessive and continuous, cannot be directly transferred to human beings. There is, nevertheless, a warning that an altered endocrine environment in human tissues might result in an abnormal expression or potentiation of growth, as in experimental animals. In fact, there has always been the suspicion that experimental animal and human tissues follow the same biological laws in this regard, but conclusive data are not available. A great difficulty in obtaining a reliable answer involves the prolonged period of latency in human beings exposed to known carcinogens. Future epidemiological studies must take full recognition of this fact.

The reference to "susceptible strains and species" and to "excessive and continuous dosage" specifically concerned MK-665 compound, an experimental Merck Sharp & Dohme oral contraceptive. It combined mestranol, an estrogen used in some marketed versions of The Pill, with ethynerone, a progestogen not used in any commercial Pill. On January 21, 1966, the company told the FDA that cancer had been found in the breasts of four of six beagles which had been sacrificed after receiving large doses of MK-665 for twelve months. The manufacturer, a division of Merck & Company, halted testing in the 467 women in whom the product was being tested. The women were put under observation. No trace of cancer was found in them.

Relatively few users and relatively small financial and other stakes being involved, the withdrawal of an experimental Pill was accomplished with comparative ease. But would there not be consequences awesome to contemplate for public officials who might try to stop the sale of marketed contraceptives which by estimate of the FDA in April 1967 were being taken by 11 million women around the world? This question was a serious one *if* a significant relation existed between MK-665 and the marketed versions of The Pill. The estrogen component, as noted, is in some marketed oral contraceptives. The progestogen component, ethynerone, differs from the progestogens in marketed mixtures in specific chemical structure. "Hence it is clearly inconsistent to consider the animal data with the new mixture to be of more significance than the huge body of pre-existing animal findings with a large variety of synthetic estrogenic compounds in numerous species of animals, including the dog," Dr. Hertz said in his appendix to the Advisory Committee report. "Either the presently marketed preparations are also to be condemned on the basis of almost certainly expectable animal findings or ethynerone should not have been condemned. The essential consideration is whether or not demonstrable carcinogenicity in animals is pertinent to the clinical problem. From a comparative physiological standpoint there is no validity in considering the recent results in dogs to be any more significant than comparable data in mice, rats, rabbits, and hamsters." The Advisory Committee concluded that to halt the testing of MK-665 was warranted. It did not suggest that halting the sale of marketed contraceptives was indicated, but it did, as reported earlier see "a warning" in the MK-665 episode.[1]

The Advisory Committee's Task Force on Carcinogenic Potential, whose members were Drs. Roger B. Scott and Hertz, urged "more extensive use of dogs and nonhuman primates in the animal testing" of oral contraceptives and in the testing of marketed versions, "if this has not been done, for mammary effects in dogs." There was no "if" about it, appalling as it is to state that fact. In the summer of 1967 Merck reported changes in the breast tissue of monkeys that had been on MK-665 for about two years—two on high dosage, and one each on medium and low dosage. The changes were said to be most likely not a precursor of malignancy. On July 5, 1967, Commissioner James L. Goddard told makers of The Pill to initiate studies of up to seven years' duration on monkeys and dogs. There was a balance of sorts: It was then seven years since the first Pill had gone on sale. A manufacturer wishing to market a new oral contraceptive now must begin long-term studies in dogs and nonhuman primates. Until July 1967 the requirement was merely for two-year studies in dogs and rats.

In the March–April 1968 issue of *CA—A Cancer Journal for Clinicians,* published by the American Cancer Society, Dr. Hertz was asked by the editor about the MK-665 episode:

[1] On March 10, 1966, the House Intergovernmental Relations Subcommittee held a hearing on the MK-665 episode at which William W. Goodrich, FDA's counsel, testified that agency regulations required Merck to report its "alarming finding" immediately. The beagles were sacrificed on July 30, 1965, but four months elapsed before tissue sections were examined under a microscope. After cancer was discovered in the tissues, on December 9, Merck spent time "getting in touch with their consultants" rather than with the FDA, Goodrich said. The agency was notified 43 days later. The company issued a statement saying it had acted "responsibly and as promptly as warranted." Goodrich testified that the 43-day delay "was a violation," and in April 1968 recommended to the Justice Department that Merck be prosecuted, but the Justice Department declined.

EDITOR: Is there any reason to believe that the results of animal studies are applicable to man?

DR. HERTZ: Yes. Pharmacologic phenomena so readily reproducible in such a wide variety of animals must be regarded as potentially applicable to man. This is especially noteworthy because, conversely, all known human carcinogens readily produce tumors in animals and sometimes in the same sites. . . .

EDITOR: In summary, then, you believe that women who use steroid contraceptives for prolonged periods run a risk of eventually developing cancer?

DR. HERTZ: Yes. There is some risk, and the extent is undetermined. . . .

Here in summary are significant points about The Pill and specific forms of cancer:

CERVICAL CANCER

In trying to find out if there is an association with The Pill, and if there is one what it is, a major difficulty is what the report of the Food and Drug Administration's Advisory Committee called "the geographic, socioeconomic, and ethnic factors of the population sampled. . . . For example, the prevalence of carcinoma in situ [precancerous cellular changes in the cervical region which can be detected with Pap smears and is most always curable] and invasive cancer in Puerto Rico was almost six times that of a metropolitan New York group composed of women, for the most part, from a higher socioeconomic level." The report emphasized that available data were inadequate and difficult to interpret, and that "any valid conclusion must await accurate data on a much larger group of women studied for at least 10 years."

The data situation began to change sharply in September 1968. On September 13 the American Cancer Society brought researchers together at Cherry Hill, New Jersey, to hear, among other things, a report about a study made by Drs. Myron R. Melamed, a pathologist at the Memorial Sloan-Kettering Cancer Center in New York City, and Hilliard Dubrow, an obstetrician who advises Planned Parenthood of New York City on cancer research. No announcement was made of the meeting, which was closed to all but

invited scientists. However, I learned of the meeting and went
there to try to find out what was in the report, which dealt
with about 35,000 clients of Planned Parenthood Clinics. The
Cancer Society's Dr. Jack Milder tried to dissuade me from
staying, in keeping with the Society's policy of closing meetings at which preliminary data are offered so that experts can
subject them to frank, uninhibited scrutiny before possible
publication. At a coffee break I was able to chat for a few
moments with a participant who was deeply concerned about
stories in general news media that could panic women. I said
that irresponsible reporting is, of course, to be criticized, but
that I had seen no comparable concern about the torrents of
promotional publicity which in a sense had panicked women
into going on The Pill in the first place. After the meeting
Drs. Melamed and Dubrow, whose work was supported with
grants from the Public Health Service, refused to be interviewed. They said they had not prepared a formal paper but
gave assurances that in due time their findings would be published. The atmosphere—tense from the time of my arrival—
finally became such that Dr. Milder told me, "You have
overstayed your welcome." I then left—but not without the
facts I needed to do a story next morning for the *Washington
Post* saying that preliminary data showed a higher prevalence
of precancerous changes in cervical tissue in users of The Pill
than in users of diaphragms, but that factors including differences in rates of sexual activity among the two groups of
women left unanswered the question whether The Pill caused
the greater prevalence. There is a rare irony about the efforts
to maintain secrecy from physicians and from women who
were on, or were considering going on, The Pill. I did not
know, and apparently the scientists at Cherry Hill did not
know, that on the very morning of the hassle *The New York
Times* already had conveyed the essentials to brokers, investors, and other readers of its financial pages. Robert Metz
said in his "Market Place" column on September 13:

> Those swinging birth control pill stocks were off pace
> again yesterday as a rumor got around that there might be
> a relationship between The Pill and uterine cancer. . . .
> The rumor evidently stemmed from discussions at a
> closed meeting of the American Cancer Society regarding
> research projects that are in an early stage of development.

The Wall Street rumor—which was actively making the rounds on the floor of the Big Board—was that there was a statistically significant relationship between the pills and cancer.

However, the studies in question are nowhere near complete enough for evaluation and observers at the Cancer Society indicated that no relationship had been established.

In a statement on November 1 the FDA's Advisory Committee said that a review of the available evidence neither confirmed nor refuted a cause-effect relation between The Pill and cervical cancer. At the same time the committee advised every woman on The Pill to have a breast examination and a Pap smear every six months or once a year. Months went by without publication of the Melamed-Dubrow study. On February 14, 1969, *Medical World News* underscored the sensitivity of the issue by saying that while the *Journal* of the American Medical Association had put "a bright red 'rush' label" on a report submitted by the two researchers, "the public relations department at Sloan-Kettering denied that any report had been written by the Melamed-Dubrow team." In Chicago an AMA spokesman told me in March that the report had been received several months earlier, had not been rejected, and had a "strong possibility of being published," provided the authors would agree to certain suggested revisions.

Meanwhile, *Medical World News* reported, another study —also considered by the FDA to be inconclusive—had shown a sixfold increase in precancerous changes in cervical tissue. This study involved 40,000 Planned Parenthood clients. Dr. George Wied of the University of Chicago, who conducted the study, was quoted as saying that it would be "at least three years before we have any answers." Dr. Wied had prepared a paper that was scheduled for publication in a University publication, *Lying-In: The Journal of Reproductive Medicine*. After the scientist received two grants totaling $1,119,000 from the Ford Foundation for further studies, publication of the paper was canceled. A University spokesman told the *Washington Post* that the grants make possible "a more comprehensive study" and that consequently the findings that had been set for publication were being "re-evaluated." The spokesman was unable to predict when the "re-evaluated" findings would be made public.

Dr. Herbert Ratner wrote an appropriate letter of congrat-
ulations to *Medical World News* and an appropriate letter of
protest to Dr. John H. Talbott, editor of the *Journal* of the
AMA, which had prominently printed an article by an official
of G. D. Searle & Company, a leading advertiser, purporting
to show that The Pill did not cause clotting. Dr. Ratner, who
in addition to teaching at Loyola University and editing *Child
and Family,* is public health director of the Village of Oak
Park, Illinois, objected to "an evolving double standard in
which what favors The Pill, including preliminary results,
gets ready publication, but what is adverse gets delayed or no
publication at all." He continued:

> It is the prescribing physician who has the ultimate ther-
> apeutic responsibility. He, therefore, has a right to all rele-
> vant information. When a reasonable doubt of safety ex-
> ists, he, pre-eminently, should know about this, to say
> nothing of his patient who has a moral and legal right to
> informed consent. What has happened to the letter and
> spirit of the Kefauver bill: that a drug be proven safe be-
> fore, not after, it is marketed?
>
> It is depressing to think that we may be entering an era
> in which scientists, editors, social engineers and others will
> determine what scientific data should or should not be
> shared by the physician responsible for the individual ther-
> apeutic decision.

Dr. Ratner wrote the letter on February 18. In June *Medical Tribune* said the *Journal* of the AMA had decided not to
publish the Melamed-Dubrow paper and quoted Dr. Melamed: ". . . we could not agree on the revisions—if that is
what they want to call them." The paper was offered to the
British Medical Journal, a publication of the British Medical
Association, which printed it on July 26. The conclusions
were in keeping with the initial report in the *Washington Post*
in September 1968. "There is a small but significant difference" in the prevalence rates of precancerous changes in cervical tissue (carcinoma in situ) in a population choosing and
using the diaphragm and a population choosing and using
The Pill, the authors said. They reported that the difference
was "consistently present" after corrections were made for
factors known to influence cervical carcinoma: age, ethnic
origin, age at first pregnancy (which reflects early sexual ex-

perience), number of live births, and family income (which reflects socioeconomic status). Again making allowance for all of these considerations, the authors said, "There is still a significantly higher rate for cervical carcinoma within the population choosing and using steroid contraceptives."

BREAST CANCER

The FDA Advisory Committee, in its 1966 report, said, "The relationship of the oral contraceptives to breast cancer in the human being is unknown. . . . There are data that give contributory, although not very strong evidence to both sides of the question." It is a universal clinical practice to prohibit use of The Pill or of substances containing estrogen in *young* women with a known breast cancer. (Paradoxically, a substantial proportion of women well past the menopause and even some younger women with breast cancer experience regression of the disease under estrogen treatment.) Advocates of The Pill, however, imply that the ability of estrogen to modify the activity of established cancer is pertinent only to patients with "pre-existing" breast cancer (the FDA labeling says The Pill should not be given to patients "with known or suspected carcinoma of the breast"). Dr. Roy Hertz, in his appendix to the committee report, calls the implication "untenable." The reason is essentially that by the time a lump can be felt in the breast cancer is well along, and surgery is usually indicated. In other words, breast cancer can be present during a very long latent period, can escape detection, and can be altered in its activity by The Pill. Further, the effects of a substance that promotes cancer of the breast do not necessarily halt when exposure to the substance stops.

Since 1896, Dr. Hertz has pointed out, there has been an accepted clinical practice for the treatment of young women with breast cancer. That practice has been to remove the ovaries, in order to suppress the growth of the tumors by eliminating a source of estrogen. But the reduction in estrogen output obtained by this drastic surgery is of the same order as the increased input of synthetic estrogen from use of The Pill.

Were cases of breast cancer being reliably reported to the FDA for processing by its giant computer? We had the assurance given by Dr. Joseph F. Sadusk, Jr., soon after he joined the agency as its top doctor that "we are not worried." He also said, for an article in the July 3, 1964, *Life*, "But we're going to watch it." Two years later Don Oberdorfer, then of the Washington Bureau of Knight Newspapers, reported the "startling" results of what the watching had produced two years later. He said that the Advisory Committee had found in FDA files "only a single case of breast cancer in a woman taking oral contraceptives." Yet, Oberdorfer said, the National Cancer Institute said that 317 cases a year normally would be expected among each one million women in the child-bearing age group. "On this purely statistical basis, the 3,800,000 women known to be taking oral contraceptives would have developed at least 1,200 cases of breast cancer last year," Oberdorfer said in a story in January 1967. "Yet the FDA had only heard of one."

It is true that although estrogens have been used clinically for more than a quarter-century, the incidence of breast cancer in women has not changed much, and extremely few cases have been reported in women on an estrogen regimen. However, Dr. Hertz said in his appendix, these data relate—almost entirely—not to young women but to women of menopausal or post-menopausal age. He cited a report by Dr. B. J. Kennedy in 1962 in *Cancer* saying, "In premenopausal women with breast cancer or in patients in whom castration [removal of the ovaries] produced a regression of tumor, there is no doubt that small physiological doses of estrogenic hormone may stimulate the growth of cancer." Dr. Hertz also pointed out that, as noted earlier, the published data on cancer incidence as of 1966 in women under 40 was limited to 85 patients. Dr. Hertz concluded:

Of course, additional data reside in the individual clinical records of numerous institutions and private offices. However, offhand generalizations from such uncontrolled clinical experience without appropriate followup is notoriously misleading. Even very extensive uncontrolled clinical accounts are not the equivalent of soundly developed epidemiological data. Our inadequate knowledge concerning the relationship of estrogens to cancer in women is comparable with what was known about the association between lung cancer and cigarette smoking before extensive epidemiological studies delineated this overwhelming significant statistical relationship. In the absence of similarly extensive studies regarding the effect of exogenous [originating outside the body] estrogens on the incidence of breast cancer in women we are ill-advised to ignore the mass of observations clearly relating both endogenous [originating inside the body] and exogenous estrogens to the pathogenesis of this disease in both man and animals.

ENDOMETRIAL MALIGNANCY

The Advisory Committee report said that endometrial carcinoma is "primarily a disease of postmenopausal women and only five to eight percent of the cases of this cancer occur before the age of 40." The data on young women, the report said, "do not permit any conclusions relative to the effect, either adverse or beneficial, of these contraceptive pills on endometrial cancer. . . . There is no evidence, at present, that these compounds are curative."

OTHER CANCERS

The Advisory Committee report said, "Malignant lesions in the pituitary, kidneys, ovaries and bone marrow have been found in animals after treatment with certain sex hormones, but at present there are no human corollaries."

134189

Mother and Child IV

FERTILITY AND STERILITY

There were the by-now-predictable pitches that initially could not be met with contrary evidence. In November 1964 *A Prescription for Family Planning,* the G. D. Searle & Company "reference for professional use," advised family-planning counselors that The Pill will not cause women to become sterile. Citing early research by Dr. John Rock and Gregory Pincus, the company said, "There is suggestive evidence, on the contrary, that fertility is increased. . . . Researchers have termed this action of Enovid the 'rebound' effect." The notion bounded into the pages of the *Journal* of the American Medical Association where on October 25, 1965, the AMA's Committee on Human Reproduction said, "It is already clear that the use of this method of contraception has no effect on future fertility after its discontinuance. Indeed, there is some evidence that discontinuation . . . is followed by a period of enhanced fertility, presumably because of a 'rebound' phenomenon." In February 1966 Dr. Alan F. Guttmacher wrote in *Good Housekeeping,* "It can be stated flatly that the pills do not interfere with a woman's ability to bear children when she stops taking them. In fact, her fertility may be increased." Taking the ball on the rebound, Dr. Edwin J. DeCosta, the Chicago obstetrician who wrote an "AMA-authorized" blurb for The Pill in *This Week,* told the Illinois Academy of General Practice in April 1966, as reported by Arthur J. Snider of the *Chicago Daily News:* "Loss of fertility—none."

In the absence of evidence, resonant declarations such as "It can be stated flatly" and words such as "none" are more appropriate to cultists than to physicians. Almost a year before these unequivocal positions were taken, Mead Johnson & Company, maker of the sequential contraceptive Oracon, sponsored a conference in San Francisco at which:

● Dr. A. L. Banks of the University of Washington told of six mothers who had borne two or more children, had stopped using The Pill, and "have been trying to conceive from two months up to thirty months."

● Dr. Robert H. Hall of the University of Utah told of eight patients who were experiencing an absence of menstruation after discontinuing The Pill and were "hoping to get pregnant."

The issue was brought squarely before the medical profession on February 28, 1966, when the *Journal* of the AMA published a report by three San Jose, California, obstetrician-gynecologists, Drs. James M. Whitelaw, Vincent F. Nola, and C. F. Kalman. In the preceding year they had treated seventeen women, most of whom were fertile before starting on The Pill, who developed irregularity in their menstrual cycles, who stopped taking The Pill, and who found themselves infertile—in some cases probably permanently. On the basis of communications with other physicians, these doctors feel there probably are "hundreds of such cases that are unreported." In a slap at Dr. John Rock, they said, "Let's be honest about The Pill"—the title of a magazine piece Dr. Rock had done—and inform women who have never borne a child and those with but one living child "of the possibility of being relatively infertile for undeterminate periods of time following discontinuation of oral contraceptives."

Later, in the May–June 1968 issue of *Fertility and Sterility,* Dr. Whitelaw, of O'Connor Hospital in San Jose, recalled that Dr. Rock and his associates, the originators of the "rebound" concept, had given Enovid to women who had been ovulating, or were fertile. Why, he asked, is it logical, then, to give The Pill to women who are inexplicably infertile on the theory that they rebound? "One is forced to ask, 'From what do they rebound?' " Indeed, he said, results in a series of 38 infertile patients treated with Enovid "do not substantiate the findings of Rock and coworkers. . . ." He went on to say:

Over the past five years 362 infertility patients were seen in the author's private practice who had been treated unsuccessfully with oral contraceptives. . . . In the light of these results, as well as the consideration that absolute sterility is induced by the oral contraceptives, and the evidence of possible deleterious effects on the ovary and menstrual cycle, oral contraceptives are contraindicated in the treatment of so-called normal infertile females. . . .

McCall's initiated and supported a survey on The Pill among members of the American College of Obstetricians and Gynecologists and in its November 1967 issue reported on the replies from 6733 (90 percent) of the specialists. The magazine said that 84 percent of the respondents reported "that some patients were unable to become pregnant when they wanted to. Almost half reported that the difficulty occurred rarely; close to a third said that it happened occasionally; and only four percent described it as frequent." Dr. P. C. Steptoe reported in the *British Medical Journal* for March 30, 1968, on an analysis of the ovarian tissue of women who had been on The Pill for three or more years. He warned that long-term use "carries with it a definite danger of producing irreversible sterility."

POSSIBLE EFFECTS ON OFFSPRING

The suppression of ovulation by The Pill, Dr. Roy Hertz has said, is an "unequivocal abnormality." What happens to the ovum that normally would have been released from the ovary: Does it die? If it survives, is it altered in any way? Dr. Hertz dealt with these questions in his appendix to the report made in 1966 by the Food and Drug Administration's Advisory Committee on Obstetrics and Gynecology.

> The only information we have now . . . is that subsequent fertilization of some ova from the same ovaries readily occurs and that a limited number of newborn derived from such pregnancies appear normal at birth. *The number of such infants thus far described in the literature is a minute fraction of that required to determine the relative frequency of congenital defects or related abnormalities of the newborn and no significant pediatric followup of these children is yet available. . . . For an adequate analysis of this problem a population of 100,000 children would be required. Moreover, the delayed clinical manifestations of many congenital abnormalities requires that these children be followed for six to nine years in order to completely ap-*

praise any possible effect upon them.[1] *It seems unjustified to assume that the suppression of the normal ovulatory mechanism of the ovary for a four-year period may not be reflected in the quality of the ova subsequently released even from an ovary in which the histological* [microscopic examination of tissue] *findings appear to be normal* [emphasis supplied].

Others have expressed concern about the genes, which are responsible for transmitting hereditary characteristics, and the chromosomes, which carry the genes. "The indiscriminate use of hormones may well rank worse in mutagenic [gene-changing] developments than will be those in the indiscriminate use of X-rays and radioactive fallouts," Dr. John A. McCluskie of Glebe, New South Wales, said in a letter in the May 13, 1967, *Medical Journal of Australia.* On October 14, 1967, in *Lancet,* Dr. David H. Carr of McMaster University in Hamilton, Ontario, said, "Chromosome abnormalities were found in six of eight abortuses [aborted fetuses] collected from women who became pregnant after an oral contraceptive. . . ." On April 26, 1968, *Medical World News* said that oral contraceptives were of "most concern" to geneticists who gathered in 1966 at the Jackson Laboratory in Bar Harbor, Maine; that the specialists were concerned that "incalculable damage" could be done before it became apparent; and that the FDA specialist studying the problem, Marvin Legator, believes that there is no greater health problem than the threat of genetic damage. His colleague, Dr. Cecil B. Jacobson, was quoted as saying, "Damage sown in the germ plasm is far more dangerous to the human race than immediate clinical complications like cancer or thalidomide, which cripple or kill a single person but are not reproduced." On October 14, 1968, Dr. David Carr reported on a study of the spontaneously aborted fetuses of 26 women who became pregnant within six months after discontinuing use of

[1] In view of such a massive absence of essential data it was ingenuous, to say the least, of Dr. Alan F. Guttmacher, president of Planned Parenthood-World Population, to tell readers of *Good Housekeeping* in February 1966, "There are no statistics to indicate that the pills have any residual effects on the embryo." There have been "no specific studies directed to this question, either," Dr. John J. Schrogie of the FDA pointed out in a speech last January 7. "The question does seem to provide ground for some realistic concern."

The Pill. Among these women the frequency of polyp-shaped growths on mucous membranes was seven times that for the fetuses of women not on The Pill. The Canadian researcher concluded that women who become pregnant within six months after halting use of The Pill have an increased risk of having a fetus which has such growths—is "polyploid"—and which will almost invariably abort. The meaning may be that "women are in some way different, presumably hormonal, for six months or more after coming off The Pill," Dr. Carr said.

Mention should be made of the finding of the Advisory Committee that superficial masculinization of the female genital tract can occur in a fetus exposed to hormonal drugs— most likely by a mother who does not know she is pregnant —in the first sixteen to eighteen weeks of gestation.

MOTHER'S MILK

In November 1966 the Food and Drug Administration, acting on a recommendation of its Advisory Committee, announced that it would require uniform prescribing instructions, or labeling, for all brands and formulations of The Pill. Up to that time a physician could look at one label and find that the product was contraindicated in a woman who was breast-feeding a child. He could look at the other labels and find a "precaution" against The Pill in lactating mothers, mainly because of the possibility of a decrease in the supply of milk.[2] The uniform labeling says:

> A small fraction of the hormonal agents in oral contraceptives has been identified in the milk of mothers receiving these drugs. The long range effect to the nursing infant cannot be determined at this time.

This ominous statement, which appears in the "warning" section of the labeling, must have come as a distinctly unpleasant surprise, especially to those who read the newspaper and wire service stories of April 15, 1966, reporting that Dr. Edwin J. DeCosta had told the Illinois Academy of General

[2] That a decrease in the milk supply occurs in a significant share of mothers on The Pill now has been recognized. Published studies include those in *Ob. Gyn. News* for December 15, 1968, *Surgery* for June 1968, and the *British Medical Journal* for September 9, 1967.

Practice that hormones are *not* excreted in the milk and "do no harm to an infant" (United Press International), or "therefore do no harm to infants" (Chicago Daily News Service). The concern of the FDA and the Advisory Committee was, among other things, with the exposure of immature gonads of male infants to the hormonal agents or to the variations of them produced by metabolic processes in the body. In animals given hormonal compounds, studies have indicated sterility in the offspring nursed by mothers that got the drugs. The Advisory Committee said:

> These compounds appear in breast milk but in minimal amounts (0.004–0.1 percent of the administered dose). Despite the small quantities of the steroids appearing in breast milk, mammary enlargement may appear in nursing infants. Administration of the androgenic steroids [hormones which control the physiologic status of the secondary sex characteristics of *males*] to newborn experimental animals at crucial periods can affect sex differentiation and behavior and result in sterility. *No data on human beings are available* [emphasis supplied].

TEEN-AGERS

For years medical scientists and a few publications, particularly the *Medical Letter,* have been concerned about use of The Pill in physically immature girls because estrogens can cause premature closure of the centers near the end of the long bones that allow growth to occur. Once these centers "close" growth is no longer possible. "I have recently seen two girls aged 13 and one aged 14 who have been given these agents for period pains," Dr. J. B. Hemsley said in the *Medical Journal of Australia* for July 3, 1965. "There are undoubtedly many others." Certainly there are; the largest single group may be girls in welfare families to whom health authorities and family-planning groups give The Pill because they are promiscuous or even because it is assumed they will become promiscuous. Until the spring of 1965 a precaution against use of The Pill in girls who had not attained their full height was in the labeling of none of the oral contraceptives. Then it was included in one. Now, however, the uniform labeling says that The Pill "should be used judiciously in young patients in whom bone growth is not complete." In April 1967 Dr. James L. Goddard, then Commissioner of the Food and Drug Administration, emphasized this precaution in the speech, mentioned earlier, to Planned Parenthood physicians in Atlanta, and at almost the same time subscribers to *Time* received the issue with the "Freedom from Fear" cover story. This told about a mother who "announced that she was already slipping The Pill into her daughter's breakfast milk." There was no mention of the particular danger to an immature girl, or of the fact that by law and by sound medical practice The Pill is supposed to be prescribed for the person using it, not her mother. On May 2, 1968, Dr. Louis M. Hellman, who is chairman of the FDA Advisory Committee but who gives the frequent impression of being less than overwhelmed by the seriousness of his responsibilities, had this exchange on the *Today Show* with Barbara Walters:

MISS WALTERS: Would you prescribe The Pill to a girl who was a virgin?

DR. HELLMAN: Well, I think if my daughter were a virgin and came to me as a teen-ager and we could talk about these things, yes, I'd prescribe The Pill for her.

MISS WALTERS: There's no more danger in that case than there is for a woman?

DR. HELLMAN: I think that the evidence is that the younger the individual taking The Pill, the safer they [*sic*] are.

If younger is safer, Dr. Hellman should be elated to know of a paper given on January 7, 1969, by Dr. John J. Schrogie, director of the Division of Research and Liaison in the FDA's Bureau of Medicine. There has been, he told the North American Conference on Fertility in Jamaica, "a definite and justified effort to include more adolescents in family planning programs. As a result of this emphasis, many younger girls, *some as young as 9 years of age,* have been started on oral contraceptive therapy." However, Dr. Schrogie was not elated: ". . . there is little information on hand that would seem to assure the safety of this particular group from conditions that might result from the use of such potent hormones. The chief concern here is about the effect of such

hormones on the immature pituitary gland and about the possibility that use of these compounds may lead to premature
closure of the epiphyses [the centers near the end of the long
bones], with consequent retardation of growth of the bones."

Other Diseases, Problems, Questions V

To describe the research and reports on every possible hazard of The Pill would neither strengthen my case—which by now has been made—nor, I think, be especially useful. But I do want to deal briefly with a few areas that for reasons I think obvious should be of interest.

SKIN

One of the several unforeseen side effects of The Pill has been a blotchy facial pigmentation. This may be a "disfiguring cosmetic and emotional problem," Air Force Capt. Sorrell Resnick, M.D., reported on February 27, 1967, in the *Journal* of the American Medical Association. Of 212 patients on The Pill, he said that sixty-one, or 29 percent, developed this condition, a drug-induced melasma that "is not as readily reversible" as the black pigmentation of pregnancy.

HAIR

The official FDA labeling for The Pill says that an association between The Pill and loss of scalp hair has been neither confirmed nor refuted. On April 6, 1968, in the *British Medical Journal,* Dr. Ronald Carruthers reported that The Pill is "contributing to the increase in numbers of young women complaining of diffuse hair loss."

HEADACHE

Numerous studies have associated The Pill with headaches. The most precise data known to me was accumulated by Britain's Council for the Investigation of Fertility Control, which since 1962 has been evaluating new oral contraceptives in clinical trials. "Vascular reactions are the most frequent and troublesome side effects," Dr. Ellen C. G. Grant reported on

August 17, 1968, in the *British Medical Journal*. "The commonest manifestation of these is headache. Whereas the incidence of headaches in women before joining the trial was 17 percent, the incidence of headaches among the same women varied from 8 to 60 percent during treatment with the oral contraceptive formulations." In an editorial the *Journal* said that headache "may in some cases be a small price to pay for freedom from the tyranny of fertility, but when it is considered that in Great Britain alone some half-million or more women will be taking the pills this year, and that with some combinations of progestogen and estrogen the incidence of headache rises above 50 percent, the total burden of pain is considerable."

DEPRESSION AND LOSS OF LIBIDO

Some users of The Pill become almost euphoric. Others become depressed. One of the physicians who early expressed informed concern about the effects of The Pill on the psyche was Dr. John R. McCain, professor of obstetrics and gynecology at Emory University in Atlanta. He reported that between May 1964 and October 1965 he found "disturbingly numerous" complications in forty-one patients on The Pill. "The psychiatric complications seem to me to carry the most serious potential," he said on October 21, 1965, in Norfolk at a meeting of District IV of the American College of Obstetricians and Gynecologists. Three of the forty-one patients "have told me that they were going to kill themselves," he said. Two of the three had been on The Pill less than two weeks and the third about four months. "The suicidal fears have disappeared in all three patients since omitting the contraceptive pills," he said. He noted that he had never before had patients who "have told me so dramatically of their fear of suicide."

The first prospective controlled study on psychiatric complications in users of The Pill was reported in November 1967 by Dr. Brenda Herzberg of the Medical Research Council in England. Preliminary results of this pilot effort showed that almost 10 percent of the 118 women taking The Pill for the first time became depressed, some to the point of requiring psychiatric treatment. The control group used mechanical means of contraception. Drs. K. J. Dennis and J. D'A. Jeffrey of Aberdeen Maternity Hospital said in *Lancet* for August 24, 1968, "At present it is probably true that depression and reduced libido associated with [The Pill] cause more women to discontinue oral contraception than any other single cause." Drs. Ellen C. G. Grant and J. Pryse-Davies of the Council for the Investigation of Fertility Control in England watched for six years a total of 797 women on one or more of thirty-four oral contraceptives. "The incidence of depression and loss of libido ranged from 28 percent . . . to 7 percent and was correlated with the balance of hormone activity in the particular Pill," the researchers reported in the *British Medical Journal* for September 28, 1968. "Two of the . . . women . . . became sufficiently depressed to attempt suicide." At the University of North Carolina Dr. Francis J. Kane, Jr., studied 139 relatively young, well-educated women on The Pill. More than half "reported adverse effects, at least one quarter of whom felt badly enough to wish to stop the drug," he said in the *American Journal of Obstetrics and Gynecology* last December 1. "Feelings of depression (34 percent), irritability (29 percent), and lethargy (23 percent) are most common, while disturbances in desire for and enjoyment of sex are somewhat less frequent. Psychotic reactions do occur, seemingly more often in patients who are known to have suffered emotional disturbances in the past."

DIABETES

"I can summarize the relationship between diabetes and The Pill in one short sentence," Dr. Robert W. Kistner says in his new book *The Pill: Facts and Fallacies about Today's Oral Contraceptives.* "There is no reason for you to worry about The Pill making you a diabetic any more than pregnancy doing the same thing." I can summarize my reaction to that in one short question: Why not consider a form of contraception that provides *less* reason for worry than pregnancy does about making you a diabetic?

The pancreas produces the insulin that enables the body to convert the foods we eat into energy or hold them in reserve in the liver. If the gland cannot produce insulin in the needed amount, sugars and starches accumulate in the bloodstream. In order to excrete excess sugar in the urine, the kidneys must absorb large quantities of water from the blood. There now has been considerable evidence—especially elevated levels of blood sugar—to indicate that The Pill activates diabetes in those women in whom it is latent.

METABOLISM

This is the process that converts food into basic elements needed by the body for energy and growth. Some investigators who have studied lipid metabolism—the conversion of fats and fatlike substances—have found a troubling pattern in "a substantial proportion" of women on The Pill, Dr. John J. Schrogie, the FDA official, said in the paper he gave on January 7. The pattern is one in which there is an increased production of certain substances—plasma triglycerides and low-density lipoproteins—*"which in general resembles the pattern found in middle-aged males who are otherwise considered to be at high risk from arteriosclerosis* [hardening of the walls of the arteries] *and related diseases,"* he said [emphasis supplied]. "Although these changes . . . have not been directly related to specific adverse effects up to now, a number of investigators have already expressed concern about the relatively long-term exposure of women to these abnormalities in metabolism." This is a deeply troubling report.

HIGH BLOOD PRESSURE

Several reports have shown an association between high blood pressure and some users of The Pill. Last February in San Francisco, a research team from Stanford University Medical Center told a meeting of the American College of Physicians about 100 women patients with high blood pressure. Fourteen were on The Pill—and had not had high blood pressure until they began to use it. After they went off The Pill for three months seven of the fourteen had normal blood pressure, four no longer required medication to control their hypertension, and three required much less medication than previously. The researchers were Drs. Myron H. Weinberger, R. Dennis Collins, and John A. Luetscher.

BUDD-CHIARI SYNDROME

This is a rare syndrome in which, among other things, there is clotting in the veins of the liver. The *British Medical Journal* in 1968 carried a report on a nonfatal case on January 6, one on a fatal case and a nonfatal case on January 27, and one on a fatal case on February 24. All of the victims had been on The Pill. "The acknowledged rarity" of Budd-Chiari Syndrome "must point . . . to The Pill being seriously implicated," Dr. Iris Krass said in the *British Medical Journal* for March 16, 1968.

Planning Other Women's Parenthood VI

This book has been directed almost entirely at women with education, with the ability to read, reason, and make choices. This book is not going to reach the illiterate and the impoverished in this country and abroad—the millions of women given contraceptives under programs financed by the Department of Health, Education, and Welfare, the Office of Economic Opportunity and the Agency for International Development. For years it has been an open secret that in some family-planning clinics The Pill is handed out with little if any regard for the examinations, warnings, and follow-ups that are supposed to be rigidly observed. Last year a Public Health Service specialist acknowledged in an interview, "It is common practice for a woman to be given a bag of Pills and told to come back in six months, and then not be seen for a year. Under these circumstances it is impossible for the detailed instructions in the labeling to be followed." All of this has troublesome implications for which only the rash would pretend to have easy solutions. "There is justification for the belief that if the power and prestige of government is placed behind programs aimed at providing birth control services to the poor," Dr. Frank J. Ayd, Jr., testified at a Senate hearing on June 15, 1966, "coercion necessarily results and violations of human privacy become inevitable." Dr. Ayd said the issue is not the sincerity of those who give assurance that there will be no coercion. "In practice, however, this is not what happens," he said. "In a physician-patient or a caseworker-client relationship there seldom is totally free choice for the patient or client. This is because the way questions are asked or a subject presented considerably influences a person's choice. It is natural for a doctor or a caseworker who favors a particular method of birth control to consciously or unconsciously convey his preference and desire by the way questions are formulated and asked." Dr. Ayd recalled that he had participated in a panel meeting at Johns Hopkins with Dr. Mary S.

113

Calderone, former medical director of the Planned Parenthood Federation of America and later director of the Sex Information and Education Council of the United States. She
"supported my position," Dr. Ayd said. "She spoke about her
extensive experience with birth control clinics and the manner in which physicians dealt with the clinic patients. She
concluded by remarking, 'Very often we may unconsciously
seduce the person away from a method she might choose.' "

Knowing what you now know about The Pill, how likely
do you think it is that such a person gives *informed* consent?
In this "era of consumer protection," Dr. Herbert Ratner said
in *Child and Family* for Spring 1968, a woman "has a right
to protection from manipulation and victimization." He continued:

> No right is more firmly established than the right of the
> patient to informed consent to a prescription whether sur-
> gical or medicinal. Knowledge sufficient for enlightened
> consent is a moral, medical, and legal right to which mal-
> practice suits testify. The classic statement of this right is
> found in Plato's laws . . . where Plato distinguishes be-
> tween the physician who takes care of slaves, and the one
> who takes care of freemen. Whereas the slave-doctor pre-
> scribed "as if he had exact knowledge" and gave orders
> "like a tyrant," the doctor of freemen went "into the na-
> ture of the disorder," entered "into discourse with the pa-
> tient and his friends," and would not "prescribe for him
> until he has first convinced him." The reader can deter-
> mine for himself whether the American woman, as patient,
> is treated as slave or free person.

Conclusion

There is a fair and obvious question to be asked, and there is no honorable escape from it: Should The Pill be taken off the market? Looked at purely as a drug, of course it should be, because it is, as Dr. Herbert Ratner has said, "the most dangerous drug ever introduced for use by the healthy in respect to lethality and major complications. It is certainly the most talented drug ever introduced in its ability to produce diverse and varied disease phenomena and systematic abnormalities in normal women." But it is more than a drug. It is a phenomenon complexly entwining the pharmaceutical industry, the social structure, foreign and domestic policy commitments, and the mystique of sexuality. At least at this time the idea of taking it off the market is utterly impractical and could well breed a bootleg market. The best course, it seems to me, is to bring out the facts about The Pill. That is the purpose of this book. I think it is a fair assumption that a woman whose education about The Pill has come from reading drug company brochures in her doctor's waiting room is likely to have one attitude toward The Pill; the woman who reads this book perhaps will have quite a different attitude.

"In the opinion of MWN's [Medical World News's] Moscow correspondent, the recent Soviet decision to mass-produce IUD's [intra-uterine devices] fits in with their generally conservative approach to medicine. 'They favor a mechanical device over a chemical one because its effects are limited to the uterus. But they do not want to miss out on something that might prove to be better, so they are proceeding cautiously in many directions. Meanwhile, the Western world is their guinea pig for The Pill.'"

—*Medical World News,* January 10, 1969

"The steroid pills violate a general medical principle. It is deemed safer to affect a target organ, in this case the uterus, tubes, or ovaries, directly, rather than to tinker with that affect through another organ, particularly when that organ is as important and complex as the pituitary gland. This master gland produces more than a dozen other chemicals and hor-

115

mones, each regulating a vital body process, such as thyroid
activity, water metabolism, and body growth."

> —Dr. Alan F. Guttmacher—in 1959, the year
> before The Pill went on sale—in his book
> *Babies By Choice Or By Chance*

". . . how far should we go, or try to go, in compounding
drugs for our society? This suggests an allied and somewhat
broader question: are we indeed trying to work with nature
or are we trying to work against and control it?
"In the world at large, with all the vast technologies and
powers now available, it would appear that man is moving
along rather complacently in the belief that he will one day
conquer nature and bring all its forces under his control. Perhaps he will. On the other hand there is evidence that he is
not controlling nature at all but only distorting it. . . . His
powers have extended so far that nature itself, formerly
largely protective, at least in the long historical or biological
view, seems to have become largely retaliatory. Let man
make the smallest blunder in his far-reaching and complex
physical or physiological reconstructions, and nature, striking
from some unforeseen direction, exacts a massive retribu-
tion."

> —Dickinson W. Richards, Nobel Laureate in
> Medicine, 1956, in *Drugs in Our Society*,
> edited by Paul Talalay and published in
> 1964 by the Johns Hopkins Press.

Postscript

On September 4, 1969, the Food and Drug Administration held a press conference to discuss a new report on The Pill by the agency's Advisory Committee on Obstetrics and Gynecology. Overwhelmingly, the substance of this 200-page document validates the warnings in this book. "The reservations of the first [1966] report appear to have been justified," Dr. Louis M. Hellman said in his "Chairman's Summary." "Concern about the immediate and long-range side effects of the hormonal contraceptives has increased as scientific investigations have uncovered a host of diverse biologic effects," he said. He told reporters, "The light is still yellow . . . meaning caution."

Nine years after The Pill went on sale the Committee was urging that well-designed studies be *"initiated* and supported to elucidate or eliminate the relation of the hormonal contraceptives and carcinoma of the breast and uterus" [emphasis supplied]. The relation of The Pill to the induction of cancer "is the major unsolved question," the consultants said. Similarly, a Committee task force on metabolic effects said that in users of The Pill "there appears to be no organ system tested that is not affected in some way," that on many organ systems there is "a multitude of effects," and that *it is not yet possible to draw definite conclusions about their* [the oral contraceptives'] *effect on the health of women and infants . . ."* [emphasis supplied]. In a perceptive editorial on September 12, *The New York Times* said, "What is even more disturbing than the blood clot problem, however, is the ignorance that exists about the long-term impact of present birth control drugs upon the health of the women who use them and of the infants they may have after ceasing to take these anti-pregnancy chemicals. . . . Indeed, the whole level of ignorance makes it appear premature to apply the adjective 'safe' to these powerful hormones."

For reasons that were by no means clear, the good sense displayed by the *Times* was not displayed earlier at the press conference by Dr. Herbert L. Ley, Jr., Commissioner of the FDA, when he began the proceeding by saying, "We believe the findings in the report are favorable. The report states, in

117

short, that the benefits of oral contraceptives both to the individual user and to society outweigh the risks involved in their use." This conclusion was no more justified by the body of the report than was the conclusion of the Johnson Administration that the disastrous Tet offensive in Vietnam was a victory for the United States. Calling a warning of the most ominous kind a cause for celebration does not make it so, just as acclaiming a military defeat as a triumph does not make it so. In response to a question, Dr. Ley was unable to cite a single scientific paper in three years that did not either establish a cause-effect relation with disease or raise questions about the possibility of such a relation. What Dr. Ley was practicing here was not medical science, but an arcane political science of bureaucratic survival.

No less strange was the conclusion reached in the "Chairman's Summary." Dr. Hellman said that the law nowhere defines safety, that the evaluation of the safety of a drug consequently "requires weighing benefit against risk," and that the risks are enumerated in the labeling — which, he failed to note, most patients never see and many doctors never read. Then came the tortured, tricky final sentence: "When these potential hazards and the value of the drugs are balanced, the Committee finds the ratio of benefit to risk sufficiently high to justify the designation safe within the intent of the legislation." A member of the Committee who asked not to be identified told me in a phone interview, "That's a legal statement; that's not a medical statement."

Readers of this book may be surprised and possibly amused to know that none other than Dr. Hellman, in the "Chairman's Summary," said that comparisons of the risks of The Pill with those of "pregnancy, cigarette smoking, and automobile accidents . . . are probably irrelevant, contributing little to evaluation of the relative risk." He also came up with a solemn, straight-faced passage in the report which made the point that "[n]either the public nor the press is well served if information is exaggerated, mitigated, or suppressed" — and then, under questioning, at last admitted that the 10 percent failure rate with the diaphragm which he had alleged in *Redbook,* on the *Today Show,* and in *The New York Times Magazine,* applied not to careful, well-motivated users, but to clinic patients.

A few aspects of the report modify or supplement material in this book. Estimating the popularity of The Pill, the report, drawing mainly on manufacturers' production figures, figured that in 1965 about one out of three American women and girls who had ever practiced contraception had used The Pill — and that in the ensuing four years usage doubled, apparently because of much wider acceptance by "older women and women of limited education." The admittedly imprecise calculation of the current number of users was 8.5 million in the United States and 10 million elsewhere.

The results of the American studies of the cause-effect relation between The Pill and clotting diseases were, as had been predicted, "in general agreement with those previously reported from Great Britain." The risk, which was said neither to persist after cessation of use nor to be increased by prolonged use, "was estimated by indirect methods to be 4.4 times that of the non-user." However, Dr. Philip E. Sartwell, who directed the study and is chairman of the Task Force on Thromboembolic Disorders, allowed for the possibility that the true rate might be higher or lower, saying that there was nothing "magic" about the 4.4 figure. One significant finding was a higher risk for users of the sequential oral contraceptives. In the studies, which were done under Dr. Sartwell's direction in hospitals in five cities, 15 cases of clotting occurred among users of sequentials as compared with none among the controls; in contrast, 52 cases were recorded among users of the combinations as against 23 among the group of matched non-users. Dr. Sartwell found "a sixfold estimated increase in the risk of both morbidity and mortality" from strokes among users of oral contraceptives. He confirmed that young women suffering from stroke while on The Pill "almost always have some warning, usually significant headache, prior to the onset . . ." He said the evidence "seems to show an association of at least borderline significance between heavy smoking and thromboembolism." At the same time, he said that the preliminary evidence, cited in this book, indicating a relation between particular blood types and the frequency of clotting episodes, "although interesting, requires further substantiation . . ."

Finally, Dr. Sartwell joined with British researchers in deriding "the main negative evidence published to date." This was the article in the *Journal* of the American Medical Association by Dr. Victor E. Drill of G. D. Searle & Company, Inc., which was a principal underpinning of the happy talk by Dr. Robert W. Kistner in his book *The Pill/Facts and Fallacies About*

Today's Oral Contraceptives and in an appearance last August on the *Today Show* which led Hugh Downs to make the incredible statement to the television audience, "So it's safe." The Drill evidence, Dr. Sartwell concluded after analyzing it, "is inadequate to show that the incidence of thromboembolism is either unaffected or reduced by oral contraceptives."

Certain other findings in the Advisory Committee report should be noted briefly. Indications were cited that The Pill increases sexual desire in the days preceding ovulation but decreases it in the second half of the menstrual cycle. The Pill also was said to seem to heighten the susceptibility to mental depression of those women who suffer from it before and during menstruation. Notably, "the lowest incidence" of depression and reduced libido was found among users on the sequentials. The Pill was indicated to cause jaundice at a rate of 1 in 10,000 users.

Surprisingly, the Committee, repudiating a warning in the existing labeling, said that no evidence has been found to confirm fears that The Pill can stunt the growth of girls who have not attained their full height. However, Dr. Hellman warned against use of The Pill in girls who have not yet begun to menstruate, because it could interfere with the proper onset of menstruation. This was hardly consistent with his statement in May 1968 on the *Today Show* ". . . that the evidence is that the younger the individual taking The Pill, the safer they [sic] are."

Commissioner Ley indicated that one result of the report probably will be abandonment of the present uniform labeling in favor of one set of prescribing instructions for the combinations and another for the sequentials. He acknowledged that no labeling intended exclusively for physicians will protect the patients of those doctors who ignore or minimize it — but he would not accept a reporter's suggestion that appropriate warnings should be required in each and every package received by the patient. Surely one casualty of new labeling will be the scientifically unwarranted distinction currently drawn as to clotting rates among British and American women. Dr. Hellman quite rightly deplored the situation in the many foreign countries which allow The Pill to be sold without prescription.

I asked Dr. Ley why the studies of possible causal relations with cancer and other diseases which were so urgently recommended by the Committee should be paid for by the taxpayers rather than by the manufacturers that have grown fat on profits from The Pill. "You can ask the most difficult questions," he replied, closing the press conference.

MORTON MINTZ

Washington, D.C.
September 1969

Appendixes

Appendix A

Ortho Pharmaceutical Corporation

RARITAN, NEW JERSEY 08869
February 1, 1967

Dear Doctor:

The Food and Drug Administration has asked us to call your attention to the fact that a claim in our recent advertising of ORTHO–NOVUM SQ * may be misleading.

In our introduction of this product to the medical profession we featured the theme, "The Most Effective Sequential," based on a comparison of pregnancy rates published in manufacturers' package inserts. The Food and Drug Administration has pointed out that such a comparison is invalid because there has been neither a direct comparative study of the efficacy of the three sequential oral contraceptives in the same population nor individual studies of the three products in population groups shown to be comparable. We are therefore discontinuing the promotional theme in question.

ORTHO PHARMACEUTICAL CORPORATION

Mead Johnson Laboratories

EVANSVILLE, INDIANA 47721
Telephone (812) 424-6441

June 30, 1967

Dear Doctor:

The Food and Drug Administration has requested that we call your attention to current medical journal advertisements for Oracon and Questran which the FDA regards as misleading.

Oracon®
The ad claims that the drug provides ". . . oral contraception with effects which closely parallel those of the natural hormonal cycle" and also contains a related slogan implying such effects are "So Close to Nature." The FDA points out that not nearly all

125

effects of oral contraceptives parallel those of the natural hormonal cycle and that some of the effects of these drugs are of
profound or undetermined nature.

The ad emphasizes the low incidence of certain less serious side
effects such as amenorrhea, breakthrough bleeding, weight gain,
etc. However, it fails to give adequate emphasis to more serious
known side effects—or adequate emphasis to the possible occurrence of thrombophlebitis, pulmonary embolism, or cerebral vascular accident.

The FDA points out that the pregnancy rates claimed in the ad
were incorrectly based on 1065 women instead of only 880, and
that the ad improperly features a pregnancy rate of 0.2 per 100
woman-years. While available data do not provide a reliable
scientific basis for a statement of true pregnancy rates, experience
reported to us shows that the unadjusted rate for all women who
were given Oracon was 2.0 per 100 woman-years. The rate of 0.2
used in the ad included only those patients who insisted that they
had adhered to the regimen.

Questran®
The FDA considers the summary of warning information in the
journal advertisement for Questran to be inadequate in that it did
not contain any information on precautions and warnings. We
have attached a revised "Brief Summary," which contains the
omitted precautions and warning information in capital letters.

We are discontinuing the ads in question, and future advertising
will incorporate the above corrections. The safety and effective-
ness of Oracon and Questran are not in question when the drugs
are used in accordance with the official package inserts.

Sincerely,

P. A. Walter, M. D.
Director
Medical Research Department

SYNTEX

January 22, 1968

Dear Doctor:

The Food and Drug Administration has asked us to call your attention to the fact that certain statements in recent advertising for our oral contraceptives, NORQUEN® and NORINYL®-1, may be misleading.

In the NORQUEN advertisement, the paragraph headed "Low incidence of side effects" emphasizes the low incidence of certain less serious side effects such as spotting, breakthrough bleeding, nausea, vomiting, and other gastro-intestinal disturbances, but fails to give adequate emphasis to the more serious known side effects such as cholestatic jaundice, rise in blood pressure in susceptible individuals, and mental depression which also occur in low incidence. Further, although a cause and effect relationship has neither been established nor disproved, the advertisement does not give adequate emphasis to the possible occurrence of thrombophlebitis, pulmonary embolism, and neuro-ocular lesions which have been observed in users of oral contraceptives.

The advertisements for both NORQUEN and NORINYL-1 state that "careful observation and caution are required for patients with symptoms or history of . . . cerebrovascular accident, psychic depression. . . ." The ads should have been more specific in stating:

Oral contraceptives should be used with caution in patients with a history of cerebrovascular accident and should be discontinued if there is a sudden partial or complete loss of vision, or if there is a sudden onset of proptosis, diplopia, or migraine, or if examination reveals papilledema or retinal vascular lesions, since these may be symptoms of cerebrovascular accident.

The advertisements disclose that careful observation and caution are required for patients with symptoms or history of psychic depression but do not specifically state that oral contraceptives should be discontinued if psychic depression recurs to a serious degree. Also, the ads fail to disclose that a decrease in glucose tolerance has been observed in a small percentage of patients on oral contraceptives.

We are modifying all future advertising to reflect these changes.

Sincerely,

Ben Z. Taber, M.D.
Medical Director

Syntex Laboratories, Inc.
Stanford Industrial Park   Palo Alto, Calif.
Telephone 307-0110

Appendix B

OFFICIAL LABELING OF THE PILL

The following labeling, which became effective for all brands of oral contraceptives produced after June 30, 1968, is the official version approved by the Food and Drug Administration except for deletion of material that is irrelevant here.

"No other drug on the market lists as many and such varied complications—testimony to the pervasive and universal action of sex hormones on virtually every cell of the body," Dr. Herbert Ratner said in *Child and Family*. "Furthermore, one must never forget that in the case of the oral contraceptives one deals not with natural hormones but with artificial or synthetic substances capable of abnormal, unpredictable, and possibly disastrous effects."

CONTRAINDICATIONS

1. Patients with thrombophlebitis, thromboembolic disorders, cerebral apoplexy, or with a past history of these conditions.
2. Patients with markedly impaired liver function.
3. Patients with known or suspected carcinoma of the breast.
4. Patients with known or suspected estrogen dependent neoplasia.
5. Undiagnosed abnormal genital bleeding.

WARNINGS

1. The physician should be alert to the earliest manifestations of thrombotic disorders (thrombophlebitis, cerebrovascular disorders, pulmonary embolism, and retinal thrombosis). Should any of these occur or be suspected, the drug should be discontinued immediately.

Studies conducted in Great Britain and reported in April 1968 [1,2] estimate there is seven to tenfold increase in mortality and morbidity due to thromboembolic diseases in women taking oral contraceptives. In these controlled retrospective studies, involving thirty-six reported deaths and fifty-eight hospitalizations due to "idiopathic" thromboembolism, statistical evaluation

[1] Inman, W. H. W. and M. P. Vessey, *British Medical Journal*, 2:193-199, 1968.

[2] Vessey, M. P. and R. Doll. *British Medical Journal*, 2:199-205, 1968.

indicated that the differences observed between users and nonusers were highly significant.

The conclusions reached in the studies are summarized in the table below:

Comparison of Mortality and Hospitalization Rates Due to Thromboembolic Disease in Users and Nonusers of Oral Contraceptives in Britain.

| Category | Mortality Rates | | Hospitalization Rates (Morbidity) |
	Age 20-34	Age 35-44	Age 20-44
Users of Oral Contraceptives	1.5/100,000	3.9/100,000	47/100,000
Nonusers	0.2/100,000	0.5/100,000	5/100,000

No comparable studies are yet available in the United States. The British data, especially as they indicate the magnitude of the increased risk to the individual patient, cannot be directly applied to women in other countries in which the incidences of spontaneously occurring thromboembolic disease may be different.[3]

2. Discontinue medication pending examination if there is sudden partial or complete loss of vision, or if there is a sudden onset of proptosis, diplopia, or migraine. If examination reveals papilledema or retinal vascular lesions, medication should be withdrawn.

3. Since the safety of [The Pill] in pregnancy has not been demonstrated, it is recommended that for any patient who has missed two consecutive periods, pregnancy should be ruled out be-

---

[3] Dr. Herbert Ratner is correct in saying that this paragraph disclosed a "deference [by the FDA] to the interests of drug manufacturers," because it raised a doubt about the relevance of the British findings for American women. Yet, when it suited their purposes, the companies did not hesitate to suggest a universal applicability of Puerto Rican data, although Commonwealth women are in significant ways less comparable to most mainland women than are British women.

Dr. Alan F. Guttmacher, president of Planned Parenthood-World Population, has implicitly conceded the validity of Dr. Ratner's complaint. On July 20, 1969, in *The New York Times Magazine,* C. P. Gilmore quoted Dr. Guttmacher: "A lot of doctors were skeptical about the British study and questioned whether its results could be transferred to this country. But the British had a singularly well-controlled and accurate study. We just couldn't write it off, *no matter how much we wanted to*" [emphasis supplied]. Would an unbiased scientist have wanted to "write it off?"

fore continuing the contraceptive regimen. If the patient has not adhered to the prescribed schedule the possibility of pregnancy should be considered at the time of the first missed period.

4. A small fraction of the hormonal agents in oral contraceptives has been identified in the milk of mothers receiving these drugs. The long range effect to the nursing infant cannot be determined at this time.

PRECAUTIONS

1. The pretreatment physical examination should include special reference to breast and pelvic organs, as well as a Papanicolaou smear.

2. Endocrine and possibly liver function tests may be affected by treatment with [The Pill]. Therefore, if such tests are abnormal in a patient taking [The Pill], it is recommended that they be repeated after the drug has been withdrawn for two months..

3. Under the influence of estrogen–progestogen preparations, pre-existing uterine fibromyomata may increase in size.

4. Because these agents may cause some degree of fluid retention, conditions which might be influenced by this factor, such as epilepsy, migraine, asthma, cardiac or renal dysfunction, require careful observation.

5. In breakthrough bleeding, and in all cases of irregular bleeding per vaginum, nonfunctional causes should be borne in mind. In undiagnosed bleeding per vaginum, adequate diagnostic measures are indicated.

6. Patients with a history of psychic depression should be carefully observed and the drug discontinued if the depression recurs to a serious degree.

7. Any possible influence of prolonged [Pill] therapy on pituitary, ovarian, adrenal, hepatic, or uterine function awaits further study.

8. A decrease in glucose tolerance has been observed in a significant percentage of patients on oral contraceptives. The mechanism of this decrease is obscure. For this reason, diabetic patients should be carefully observed while receiving [Pill] therapy.

9. Because of the effects of estrogens on epiphyseal closure [The Pill] should be used judiciously in young patients in whom bone growth is not complete.

10. The age of the patient constitutes no absolute limiting factor, although treatment with [The Pill] may mask the onset of the climacteric.

11. The pathologist should be advised of [Pill] therapy when relevant specimens are submitted.

ADVERSE REACTIONS

A statistically significant association has been demonstrated between use of oral contraceptives and the following serious adverse reactions: thrombophlebitis, pulmonary embolism.

Although available evidence is suggestive of an association, such a relationship has been neither confirmed nor refuted for the following serious adverse reactions: cerebrovascular accidents, neuro-ocular lesions, e.g., retinal thrombosis and optic neuritis.

The following adverse reactions are known to occur in patients receiving oral contraceptives: nausea, vomiting, gastrointestinal symptoms (such as abdominal cramps and bloating), breakthrough bleeding, spotting, change in menstrual flow, amenorrhea during and after treatment, edema, chloasma or melasma, breast changes: tenderness, enlargement and secretion, change in weight (increase or decrease), changes in cervical erosion and cervical secretions, suppression of lactation when given immediately postpartum, cholestatic jaundice, migraine, rash (allergic), rise in blood pressure in susceptible individuals, mental depression.

Although the following adverse reactions have been reported in users of oral contraceptives, an association has been neither confirmed nor refuted: anovulation post treatment, premenstrual-like syndrome, changes in libido, changes in appetite, cystitis-like syndrome, headache, nervousness, dizziness, fatigue, backache, hirsutism, loss of scalp hair, erythema multiforme, erythema nodosum, hemorrhagic eruption, itching.

The following laboratory results may be altered by the use of oral contraceptives (see sections on clinical laboratory): hepatic function—increased sulfobromopthalein and other tests; coagulation tests—increase in prothrombin Factors VII, VIII, IX, and X; thyroid function—increase in PBI, and butanol extractable protein bound iodine and decrease in T^3 values; metyrapone test; pregnanediol determination.

Glossary

Amenorrhea: absence of menstrual periods.

Anovulation: cessation or suspension of release of an ovum.

Breakthrough bleeding: bleeding that occurs *while* The Pill is being taken.

Carcinogen: a substance that causes cancer.

Carcinoma: cancer derived from the lining cells of organs.

Cerebrovascular: pertaining to the blood vessels of the brain.

Chloasma: brownish discolorations of the skin, such as often occurs in patches in pregnancy.

Cholestatic jaundice: yellowness of the skin and eyes caused by a blockage of the bile ducts of the liver which results in bile pigments accumulating in the blood.

Climacteric: the menopause.

Contraindications: medical conditions in which a drug should not be used.

Cystitis: inflammation of the urinary bladder.

Diploplia: double vision.

Edema: swelling or bloating of body tissues.

Embolus (pl. *emboli*): A piece of a clot, or thrombus, that has broken off and traveled to another site in the body.

Endocrine glands: glands of internal secretion that release substances into blood or lymph systems; the substances then stimulate other organs.

Endometriosis: a condition in which bits of the tissue that line the womb spread via the Fallopian tubes to the pelvic organs and there, each month, function as mini-wombs.

Epiphyses: centers near the end of long bones that allow growth to occur; when these centers "close," growth is no longer possible; estrogens can cause premature closure. (epiphyseal, *adj.*)

Erythema multiforme: an acute, inflammatory skin disease.

Erythema nodosum: an eruption, usually on the front surfaces of the legs below the knees, of crops of tender nodules varying in color from pink to blue.

Estrogen: female sex hormone produced by the ovaries responsible for development of secondary sexual characteristics and cyclic changes in the uterus; the estrogens used in The Pill are produced synthetically and are not identical to those produced in nature.

Fibromyomata: benign tumors of the womb composed of muscle and fibrous tissue.

Hermorrhagic: pertaining to an escape of blood from the blood vessels.

Hirsutism: excessive growth of hair.

Hormone: a secretion of an endocrine gland; produced synthetically for The Pill. (hormonal, *adj.*)

Hypermenorrhea: excessive menstrual flow.

Idiopathy: a primary disease of spontaneous origin. (idiopathic, *adj.*)

Lesion: a change in tissue structure caused by disease or injury.

Melasma: brownish discolorations of the skin, such as often occurs in patches in pregnancy.

133

Migraine: severe headache on one side of the head, often associated with nausea, vomiting, and spots before the eyes.

Neoplasia: formation of new tissue; formation of tumors.

Neuritis: inflammatory lesions of a nerve or nerves.

Neuro-ocular: pertaining to nerves in the eyes.

Papanicolaou smear (Pap test): a test for cancer of the cervix or uterus in which cells are scraped or taken with a suction device from the mouth of the womb.

Papilledema: swelling of the optic nerve in the back of the eye.

Progesterone: a female sex hormone that prepares the lining of the womb for implantation of the fertilized egg.

Progestogen: a synthetic progesterone that, in The Pill, is combined with an estrogen.

Proptosis: a falling downward.

Pulmonary embolism: obstruction of an artery of the lung by a blood clot that has traveled through the body from the distant site where it was formed.

Renal: Pertaining to the kidneys.

Thromboembolism: blocking of a blood vessel by a blood clot that has broken away from the site where it was formed elsewhere in the body.

Thrombophlebitis: inflammation of a vein causing formation of a blood clot within the vein.

Thrombosis: the formation of a clot of blood (thrombus) within the heart or blood vessels. (thrombotic, *adj.*)

Thrombus: A clot that forms in a blood vessel.

Index

135